beautiful pilates

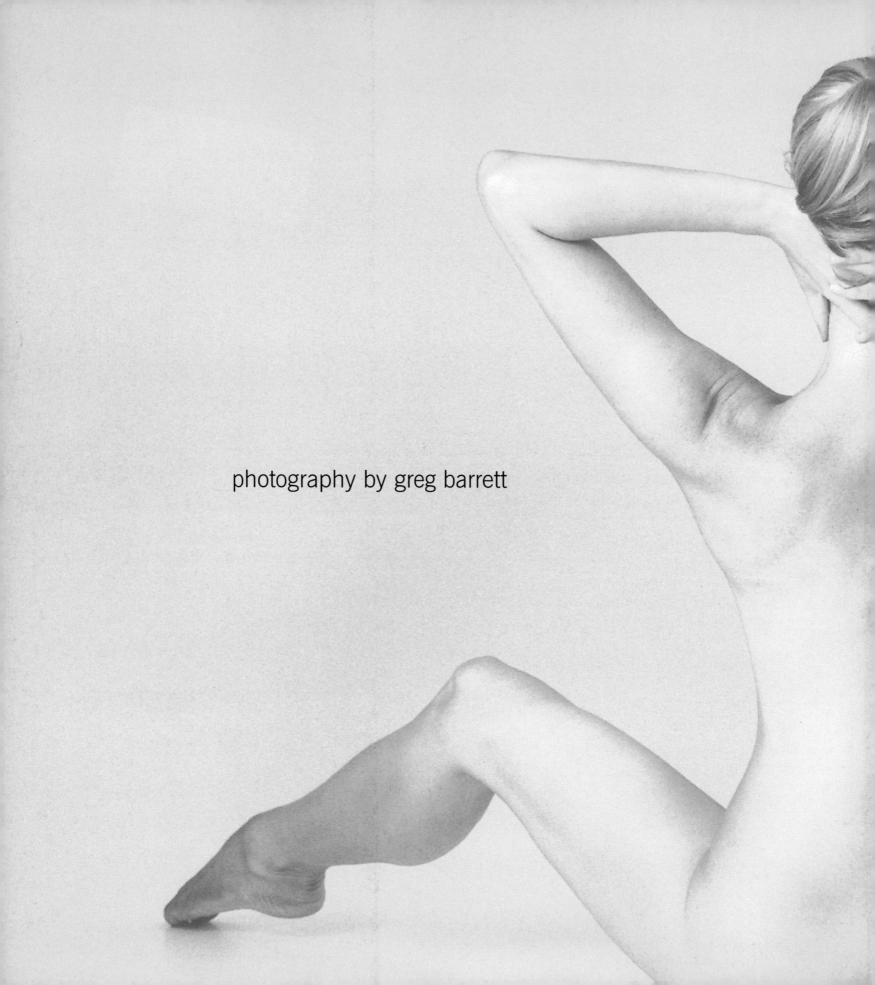

photography by greg barrett

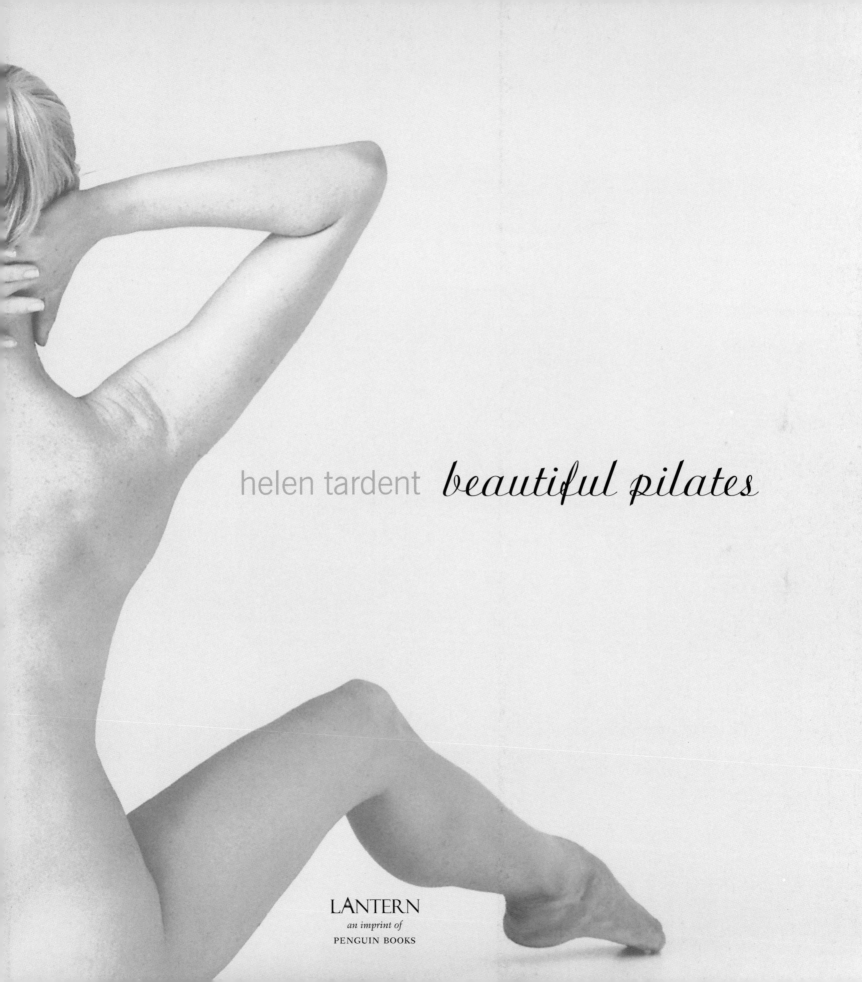

helen tardent *beautiful pilates*

LANTERN
an imprint of
PENGUIN BOOKS

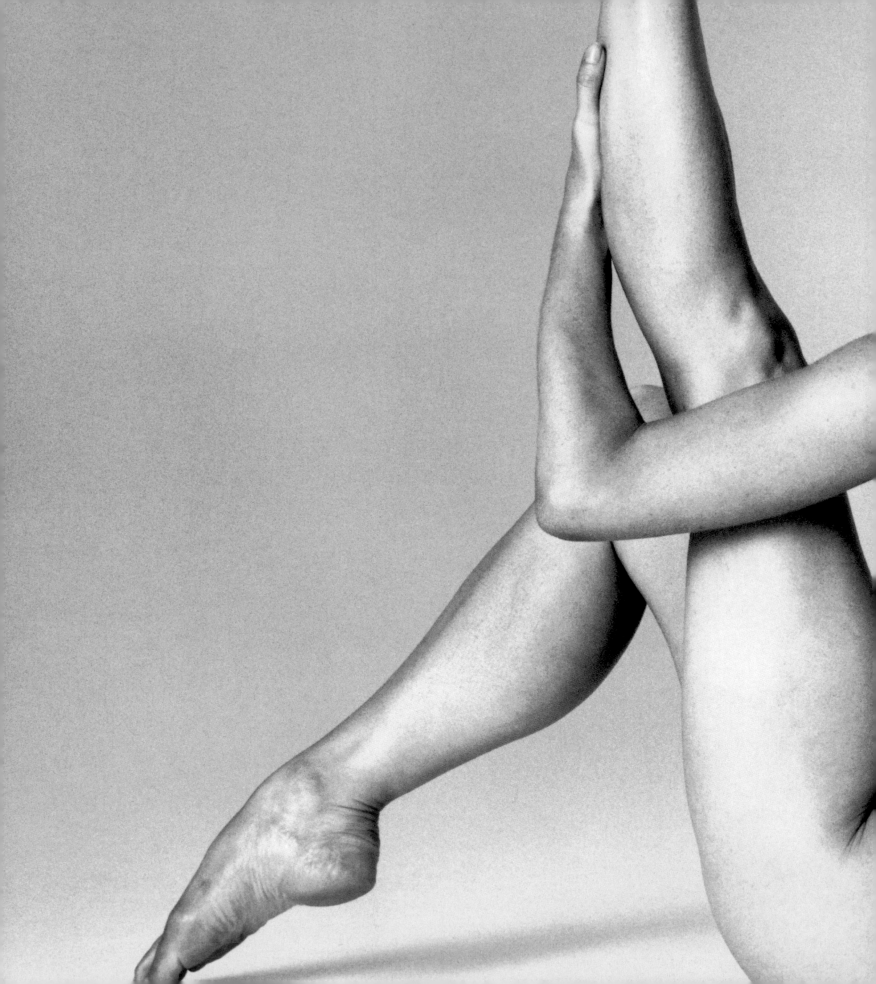

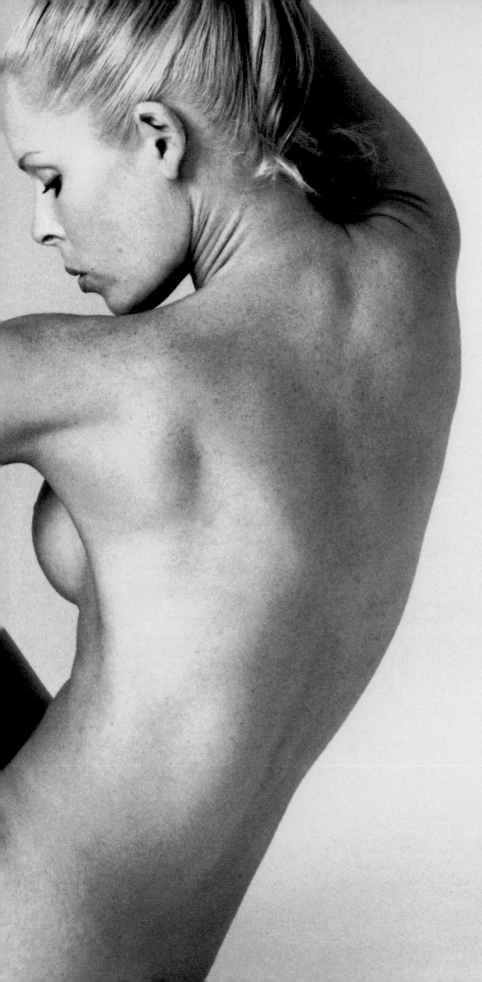

contents

For Rael Isacowitz, Sandy Sellers and Stan Barnes

history in the making

The exercise method created by Joseph H. Pilates enables you to experience the ultimate control over your mind and body, leaving your mind invigorated, your body rejuvenated and your soul content.

Our life's work is made up of myriad steps before we reach our ultimate goals, and along the way we are influenced by our families, friends, teachers, colleagues and the wider community. I am constantly inspired by the remarkable people I meet every day. These people are all around us; in fact, these people are you. We are creating new history every day. Just as Joseph Pilate's heritage and upbringing influenced his profound theories and approach to exercise and lifestyle, we are influenced and learn from his legacy.

Very limited film footage of Joseph Pilates is available; this footage, plus photographs and his two published works, *Your Health* (1934) and *Return to Life Through Contrology* (1945), are the only legacy left behind by Joseph to give us an insight into his personal philosophy and vision.

We know that he was born Joseph Hubertus Pilates in 1880, in Monchengladbach, a small town near Dusseldorf, Germany. His father was a prize-winning gymnast and his mother was a naturopath, and it is likely that both parents (and their professions) set the foundation of his theories that combine the perfect balance between the mind and body.

As a child Joseph suffered from asthma, rickets and rheumatic fever. By his early teens, however, through determination and self-discipline he had worked to overcome his physical limitations by strengthening his body and becoming an accomplished sportsman. He studied Eastern and Western forms of exercise, including Yoga, martial arts, Zen philosophy, and Greek and Roman practices. By age fourteen he had mastered diving, skiing, gymnastics and bodybuilding, and was used as a model for anatomy charts. Around this time Joseph's interest in the human body was furthered when he was given an old anatomy book by his family doctor, which he studied passionately. After age fourteen Joseph received no further formal education; his upbringing and personal study moulded his future beliefs.

Joseph moved to England in 1912 at the age of thirty-two in order to avoid the German military draft. In England he earned his living as a boxer, circus performer and self-defence instructor.

In 1914 as World War I broke out, Joseph, along with other German-born citizens, was interned in a facility in Lancaster as an 'enemy alien'. It was here that he started to develop the Matwork regime that we now know as Pilates Matwork. Further into the war Joseph was transferred to an internment camp on the Isle of Man, where he assisted in rehabilitating injured internees. By using bed springs, he designed resistance and strengthening exercises to help the bedridden internees, and the beds he reconfigured were the genesis for the Universal Reformer used in Pilates apparatus work today. Joseph later boasted that because of his exercise regime, none of his fellow internees fell victim to the deadly influenza that killed thousands of people in England in 1918.

In the early 1920s Joseph returned to Germany, where he worked for the Hamburg Police as a self-defence and fitness instructor. Around this time he met Rudolf von Laban, a dancer, choreographer and the inventor of dance notation known as 'Laban notation'; and Mary Wigman, a student of Laban's and the creator of 'Expressionist Dance'. Von Laban and Wigman were instrumental in shaping the future of the next generation of dancers, and they incorporated some of Joseph's Matwork exercises into their work. For Joseph, Von Laban and Wigman would represent the beginning of his long association with the dance community.

In 1925, after being invited (and declining) to train the new German Army, Joseph emigrated to the United States. On the long ship journey he met his future wife, Clara. Clara was a nursery and kindergarten teacher who was suffering from arthritic pain, and during the voyage Joseph shared his theories and exercises with her, using the rehabilitative aspects of his work to assist her with her pain management, and creating a personal and professional bond that would continue for more than forty years.

Joseph and Clara settled in New York, where in 1926 they opened a fitness centre called Contrology – this was also the name Joseph had chosen for what we now know as Pilates – where they worked side by side with their clients. Contrology was the basis for the contemporary Pilates studio in which Joseph's apparatus and Matwork are now taught. Contrology was housed in the same building as the New York City Ballet, and this close proximity encouraged the strong relationship between the dance community and Pilates that is still thriving today. Every major dance company and dance training facility in the world now has its own Pilates studio or one to which it is closely linked.

Although Joseph taught people from all walks of life, he became a friend and teacher to many of the great dancers and choreographers of his time. George Balanchine, the legendary choreographer who founded the New York City Ballet in 1948, studied with Joseph and consequently sent many of his dancers to classes for lengthening, strengthening and rehabilitation. Martha Graham, the creator of the contemporary dance technique the 'Graham technique', also encouraged her dancers to supplement their dance training with Contrology. Joseph trained and compared notes and philosophy with other dancers and choreographers such as Ted Shawn, Ruth St Denis, Jerome Robins and Hanya Holm, all significant for their creative flair that helped develop the world of dance that we know today.

Although Joseph's work was based around the attainment of supreme health and physical strength, he also believed that fitness should complement a broader approach to life and its rich goals. Joseph's ideals about the unity of the body and mind embodied his learning as a youth and his realisation as an adult.

In January 1966 a fire swept through the building housing Contrology. Joseph, then aged eighty-six, fell through burnt floorboards when he arrived at the scene and was trapped for some time before being rescued by fire-fighters. The effects of the smoke inhalation were considered the major contributing factor towards his death from pneumonia in October the following year.

Clara Pilates continued to manage the studio with long-time assistant Hannah Sakmurda. In 1970 Clara appointed Romana Kryzanowska, a former dancer who had studied at the Contrology studio in the early 1940s, as director of the studio. Clara remained involved in the studio until she died in 1977; Romana teaches and trains new instructors to this day.

The assistants trained by Joseph are today known as the Elders. Only two of these students, Carole Trier and Bob Seed, went on to open their own studios during Joseph's lifetime. Trier opened her studio with the blessing of Clara and Joseph. Bob Seed's relationship with Joseph, however, was not so amicable. Seed opened a studio near Contrology and attempted to solicit some of Joseph's clients. Joseph allegedly stormed over and threatened Seed at gunpoint, ordering him to leave town immediately. Seed was never seen in New York again. Just prior to Joseph's death in 1967, another two of his students, Kathy Grant and Lolita San Miguel, were awarded degrees to teach Pilates by the State University of New York, and it is alleged they were the only Elders to be officially 'certified' by Joseph. The other Elders were Eve Gentry and Bruce King, who both died in the early 1990s, Ron Fletcher, Mary Bowen and Robert Fitzgerald.

Today those who have the opportunity to work with any of the Elders will not only practise Joseph's original exercises, but will experience each individual teacher's interpretation of his work, which has evolved with every client with whom they have worked. Joseph was the ultimate entrepreneur, and as much as he is our history, today we continue to develop his original work with new research and findings in exercise and wellbeing, creating further history for the future.

the what, wear, when and how of pilates

The beauty of Pilates Matwork is that you can practise it anywhere and at any time. Choose a space that is quiet and tranquil. Have a bath-size towel handy, and if the ground or floor is hard, invest in an exercise mat that is comfortably longer than the length from the tip of your head to the base of your buttocks. Ensure you have plenty of room to move by lying on your back and swinging your arms and legs away from your body as if you were making a snow angel; if you touch an object during this test, reposition yourself until you find the ideal space.

Wear comfortable clothing that permits you to move your limbs with complete freedom, and allow yourself the luxury of bare feet.

Pilates has been used for fitness and rehabilitation since its conception in the early twentieth century. If you have any restrictions or injuries, individual attention is essential for time-effective recovery. Firstly, consult your treating medical practitioner before attempting the exercises in this book. Your physician will understand your medical history and can give you sound advice on the best approach to strengthen, lengthen and stabilise your body.

A range of Pilates exercises is ideal for women during pregnancy; however, before starting or continuing any exercise regime, consult your treating practitioner. If you are given the all clear, I recommend that you only work under the experienced supervision of a fully qualified teacher in a studio setting. There are only a few Matwork exercises appropriate during pregnancy; a combination of Matwork and apparatus exercises is ideal, and a personalised mat routine can be prepared for you to supplement your studio workout at home.

For fitness and that 'body beautiful', I recommend the invaluable experience of being personally supervised at least once a week. Think of this book as a tool for increasing your depth of understanding and inspiring you to reach greater levels of body awareness, fitness and graceful beauty.

And remember, Pilates is for everyone. Work within your own ability, without judgement, revelling in each moment you learn something new and profound about your body and spirit. We are all unique in our abilities and passions, and this is what makes our personal journeys so exquisite and beautiful.

As a beginner, keep your gains simple and rewarding. Structured breathing enhances the benefits of each exercise, but I recommend that you focus on your technique and application before adding the breathing rules. Remember that in practising the exercises you are learning a new skill, but breathing is something we do naturally every day, so allow yourself the indulgence of incorporating the breathing rules as you master the movements. When you feel comfortable with the technique of each exercise, slowly apply the breathing rules.

Pilates Matwork can be physically exhausting, so if you must eat before you exercise, ensure it is only a light snack. Exercising on a full stomach is very uncomfortable, so try to leave at least two hours between eating and exercising. You will learn very quickly the hard way if you over-indulge in food before you exercise!

Pilates Matwork can be practised every day and at any time. In the early morning Pilates stretches you and energises you for the day ahead; in the afternoon Pilates refocuses you to complete the day with clarity and direction; and in the evenings Pilates restores your sense of serenity after a jam-packed day, preparing you for a calm and peaceful end to your day. Be prepared to spend an hour on your workout. As a beginner your workout pace will be very slow and controlled, and as you progress to the more advanced levels your pace should naturally increase with your advancing skill.

Joseph Pilates believed that in order for any of us to achieve true flexibility of the body, our muscles must be uniformly developed, and as part of this philosophy he chose to combine strength and flexibility training by incorporating full range of movement through related joints in his exercise regime, rather than static stretches held for a length of time. This is why we feel so limber after a Pilates workout.

Movement is a language we express through our bodies just like talking, laughing and crying. As a dancer I have had the privilege of experiencing language through movement on the stage, in a dance studio and in everyday life. My gift to you in this book is the awareness of the unlimited potential of your body and my personal interpretation of the Pilates exercises.

Each Pilates exercise in this book includes an abstract photograph depicting the essence of the exercise. The position of my body in these abstract photographs is not necessarily part of the exercise; it is a way of expressing the body's movement and grace within the exercise.

Each exercise has a focus, imagery and precaution that relates to the exercise's specific goals. We all learn in a unique way, so as you work through this book you will notice cues from the imagery or text that will help you visualise your aims. Choose your own descriptive journey.

The Matwork is only a small part of what you can experience in Pilates. A fully equipped studio includes apparatus such as the Reformer, Cadillac, Wunda chair, Ped-o-Pull, High Barrel, Spine Corrector, Baby Arc, Magic Circle and modern apparatus that challenge your strength, flexibility, coordination and control.

My personal introduction to Pilates was word of mouth through fellow students at The Royal Ballet School in London. After retiring from ballet I returned to Australia and began teaching Pilates. Introducing Pilates to the public has been my most satisfying achievement. This book has been written for you. I hope you take as much pleasure in the beauty of Pilates as I do.

the six exercise principles of the pilates method of exercise

The Pilates Method of Exercise is a low-impact workout that invigorates the mind and elevates the spirit. Goal-specific and time-effective, the Pilates Method is a full-body workout that is ideal for any level of fitness. Pilates is often referred to as the 'thinking person's workout', encouraging you to harmoniously stimulate your brain and body. The focal point of this book is the Matwork, which is only one part of this unique method of exercise developed by Joseph Pilates. The beauty of the Matwork is that you can practise it anywhere at any time, utilising your body as resistance. With diligence you will develop strength, increase flexibility, and attain the grace and poise of a finely tuned athlete.

Every exercise designed by Joseph Pilates is governed by six underlying principles: Concentration, Control, Centring, Precision, Flowing Movement and Breathing. As you begin to master the exercises, you will notice a change not only in your posture but also in the way you move. Your body and mind will be subconsciously applying the six principles into your everyday life, the Pilates way. It is very important that you understand exactly what each of these principles represents.

concentration Every movement our body makes starts from our mind. By concentrating wholly on every detail in each exercise and practising them precisely, you will not only attain grace and suppleness but will feel your muscles working harder than they ever have before. You will also allow your mind to breathe, giving it a break from your everyday stresses, leaving you revitalised, relaxed and focused.

control It is vitally important to learn to control not only your mind, but also your body. Each exercise should be undertaken slowly and carefully to achieve a strong foundation for your body. Having total control over your body reduces your risk of injury caused by sloppy, careless movements. When practising Pilates exercises, speed is a harder skill to master. As you gain experience and learn the correct technique, you will find yourself able to quicken your pace with control, further challenging your stability and balance.

centring Think of drawing your navel to your spine, lifting your pelvic muscles or trying to do up jeans that are a size too small. These are examples of the many ways we can connect with our centre or, as Joseph called it, our 'powerhouse'. Drawing our navel to our spine not only makes us appear slimmer but has a functional use too: we now know that our pelvic floor muscles and deep abdominals have the same nerve supply, and our deep abdominals play a vital part in supporting our torso and protecting our back. So, finding your centre will take the load off your extremities (arms and legs), giving you more stamina to finish each exercise calmly and tranquilly.

precision Our greatest athletes are masters of precision. When the difference between winning a gold rather than silver Olympic medal is at stake, the athlete who is able to move through space with the least amount of excess movement, streamlined and pure in technique, will have the advantage. The grace and composure of a finely tuned athlete is due to years of disciplined training and hard work. We all admire their elegance and efficiency of movement. By carefully and precisely following the instructions in this book, you too can achieve poise and refinement.

flowing movement There are three chiefly acknowledged ways to increase flexibility: static stretching, ballistic stretching and range-of-movement stretching. Joseph Pilates favoured range-of-movement stretching combined with strength work to achieve effective results. Every Pilates exercise correctly performed is fluid and graceful, though range-of-movement stretching can be very deceptive if you are used to holding a static stretch, because your body has been conditioned to thinking that the word 'stretch' means you must hold a static pose for some time. After your first Pilates workout, take note of how limber and agile you feel.

breathing Joseph Pilates believed that by inhaling and exhaling completely, the body is revitalised with fresh oxygen and energy. In everyday life, the ideal way of breathing is to allow your lungs to fill with oxygen without any restrictions, your torso rising and falling. During structured exercise such as Pilates, or when you are lifting and carrying objects, it is very important that you keep your navel drawn to your spine and that you breathe into the back of your lungs and the sides of your ribs, to support your lower back. The breathing rules assigned to each exercise in this book enhance the benefits of the exercise, though I suggest that if you are a beginner, you leave the breathing rules until you have mastered the exercise you are performing.

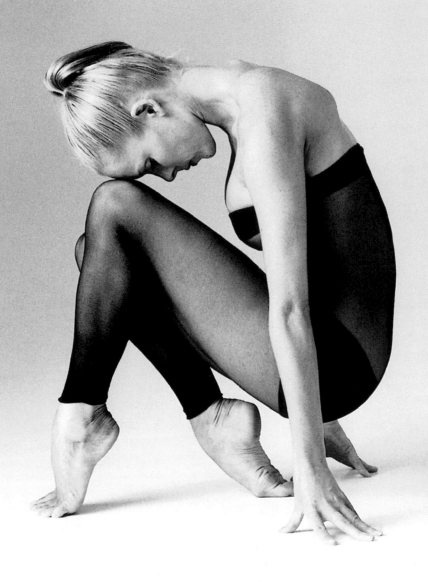

concentration

concentrate /ˈkansen,trert/ *v. & n. —v.*
1 intr. (often foll. *by on, upon*) focus all
one's attention or mental ability.

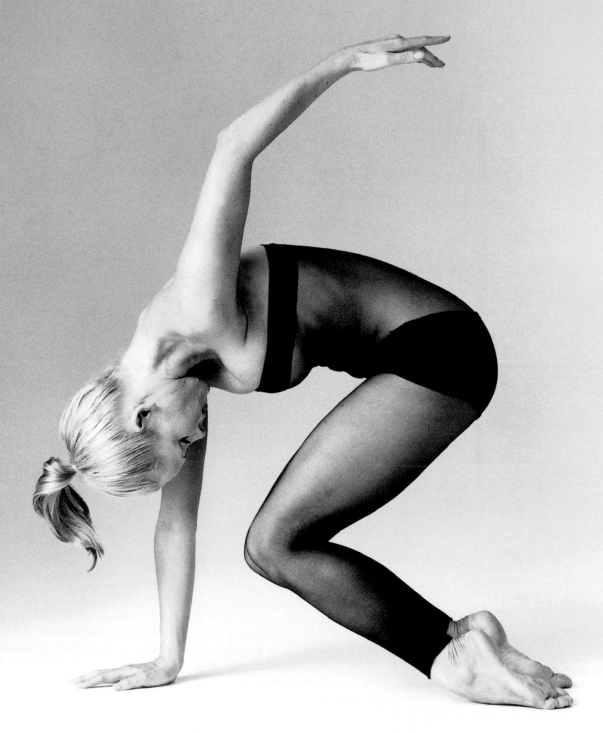

control

control /kənˈtrəʊl/ *n. & v. —n.*
1 the power of directing, command
(*under the control of*).

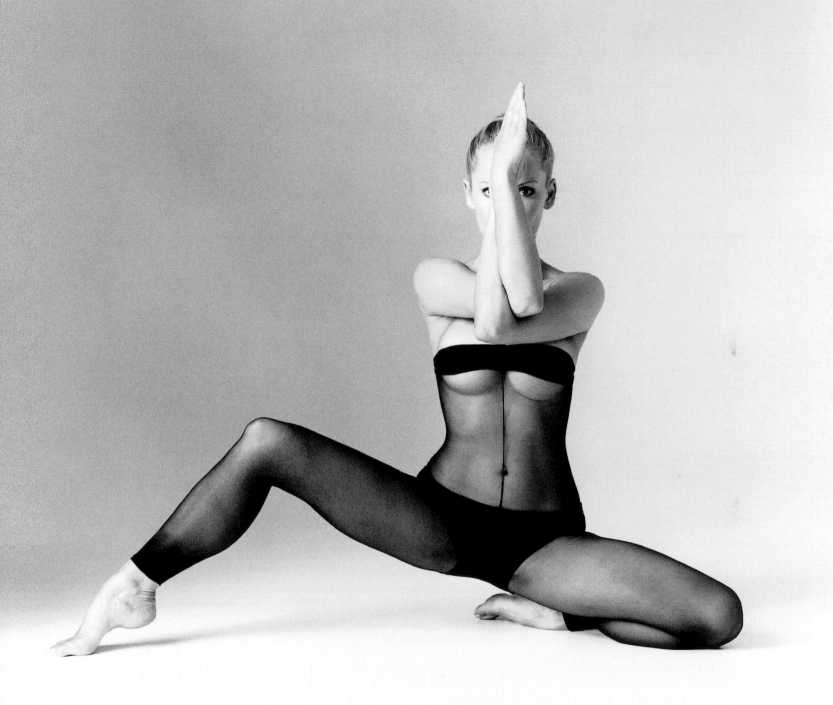

centring

centre /'sente(r)/ *n. & v.* (*US* **center**) —*n.* **1** the middle
point, esp. of a line, circle, or sphere, equidistant from the
ends or from any point on the circumference or surface.

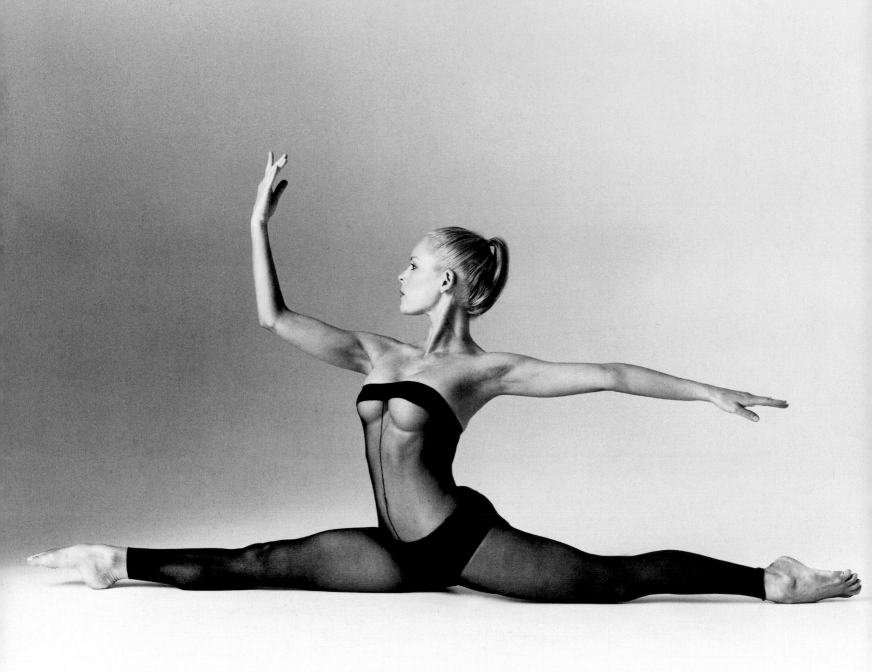

precision

precise /pri'sais/ *adj.* **1 a** accurately expressed. **b** definite, exact. **2** punctilious; scrupulous in being exact, observing rules, etc. **3** identical, exact (*at that precise moment*).

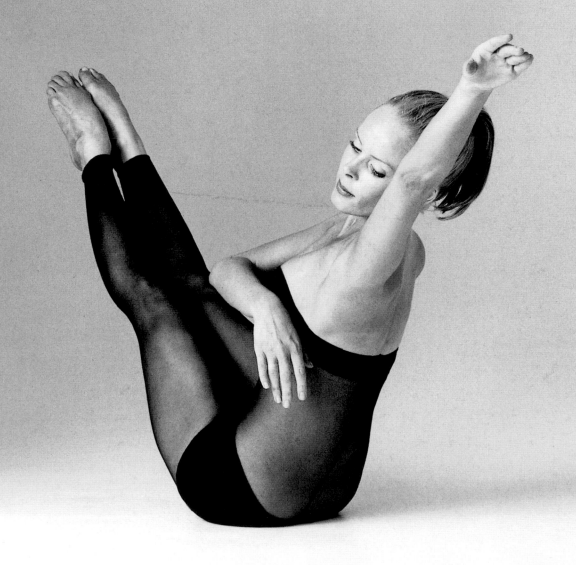

flowing movement

flow /fleʊ/ *v. & n.* — **flow chart 1** a diagram of the
movement or action of things or persons engaged
in a complex activity.
move /muːv/ *v. & n. v.* **1** *intr. & tr.* change one's
position or posture, or cause to do this.

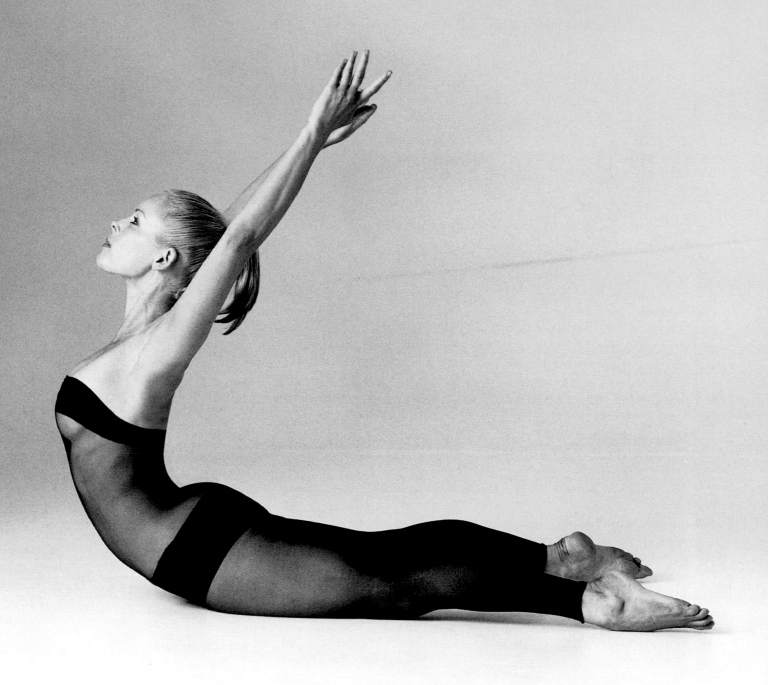

breathing

breathing /ˈbriːɔɪn/ *n.* **1** the process of taking air into and expelling it from the lungs.

For a full-body workout and maximum results, use the following exercises in the sequences shown. Remember that it is very important to work within your individual physical ability. The exercises are listed in an order that relates to your level, rather than the order that appears in the descriptive text.

Traditionally, many of the Pilates Matwork exercises are at the advanced level. In a studio setting we have many breakdowns of the original exercises to bridge the gap between each level: beginner **b**, intermediate **i**, advanced **a** and super-advanced **s**. Read the instructions carefully, ensuring that you are practising the correct variation for your level.

Build your strength, flexibility and coordination slowly and carefully, savouring every moment of your journey forward. I highly recommend you spend some time with an accomplished teacher before beginning the exercises in this book. We are all unique and beautiful beings, so what may work for you will simply not do for your neighbour. By starting your Pilates regime with a fully qualified Pilates practitioner you have the advantage of their expertise to assess your skills and abilities and give you sound advice for the future.

Your workout need take no more than a quality hour of your day. In our busy lives the time we spend on different and varied tasks should be goal-specific and time-effective. Plan ahead, because the time you spend on your body is an investment in your future.

Consult your Pilates practitioner for advice on the best time to commence each level of difficulty. Be open to your teacher changing the exercise order a little to cater for your personal needs, remembering that you are one of a kind.

The beginner and intermediate workouts offer you one workout option. The advanced and super-advanced workouts offer you two choices of workout, allowing you to keep your workouts time-effective and interesting. Give yourself five to ten weeks on each workout at the appropriate level. Rotate the advanced workouts until such time as your teacher feels you are ready for new moves.

Some exercises include a modification, which will make the exercise easier if you have an injury or restriction. I have also included variations to some exercises, either at the same level or the next level up.

Be sure to thoroughly read 'The What, Wear, When and How of Pilates' (page 4) before beginning the moves.

BEGINNER

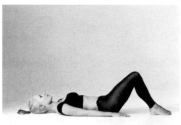

the neutral pelvis & neutral spine,
p36 >

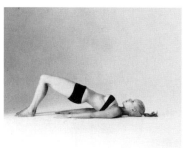

breathing, p38 >

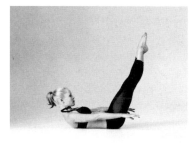

the pelvic roll-up, p41 >

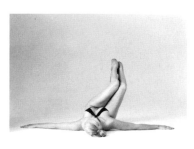

the side to side, p44
and the thoraco lumbar stretch, p44 >

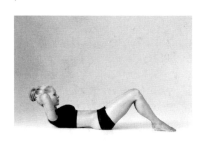

preparation for abdominals, p46 >

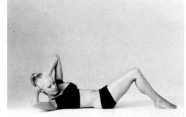
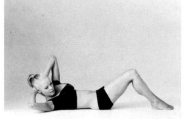
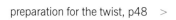

preparation for the twist, p48 >

preparation for the hundreds, p50
and the hundreds, p55 >

the roll-up, p59 >

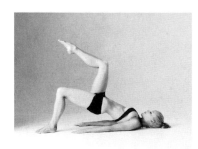
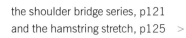

the shoulder bridge series, p121
and the hamstring stretch, p125 >

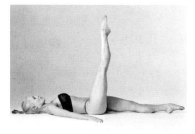

the leg circles, p67
and the lunge stretch, p69 >

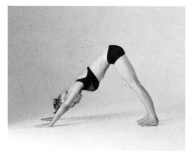

the up-stretch, p157 >

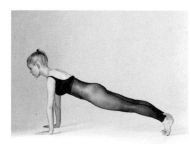

the leg pull front, p160 >

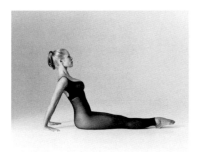

the leg pull back, p163   >

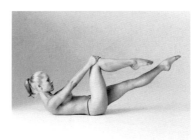

rolling like a ball, p71   >

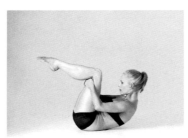

the single-leg stretch, p74   >

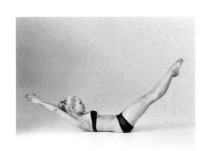

the double-leg stretch, p76   >

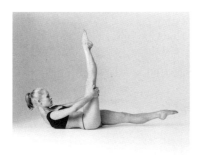

the hamstring pull, p78   >

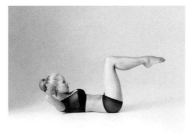

the double-leg lowers, p80   >

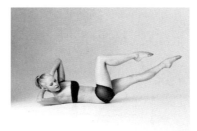

the single-leg stretch twist , p82   >

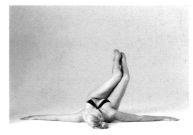

the side to side, p44   >

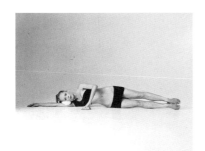

the side lifts, p133
and the quad stretch, p135   >

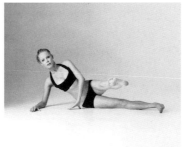

the side kick i, p137   >

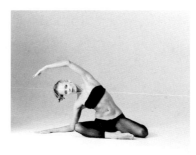

the mermaid, p176   >

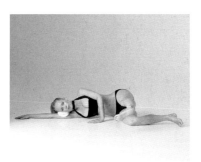

the leg lifts, p141
and the buttock stretch, p143   >

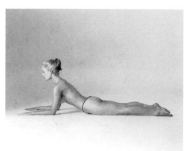

the swan dive, p101   >

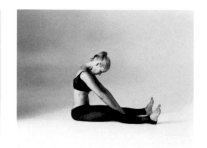

swimming, p154   >

the rest position, p108   >

the spine stretch, p85   >

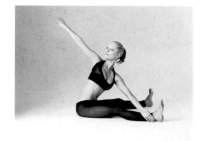

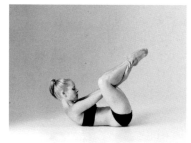

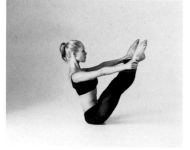

the saw, p98   >

the open-leg rocker, p89   >

the seal puppy, p183

INTERMEDIATE

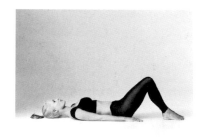

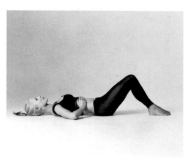

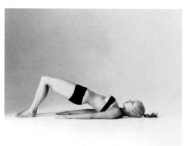

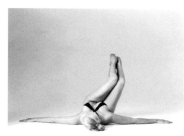

the neutral pelvis & neutral spine,
p36   >

breathing, p38   >

the pelvic roll-up, p41   >

the side to side, p44   >

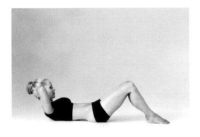 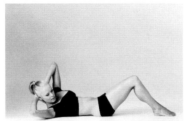 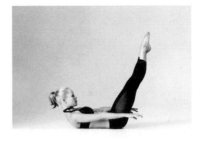 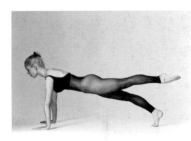

preparation for abdominals, p46   >   preparation for the twist, p48   >   preparation for the hundreds, p50   the roll-up, p59   >
                                                                              and the hundreds, p57   >

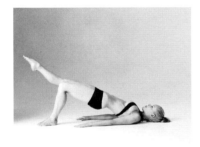 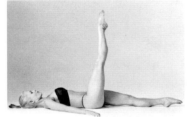 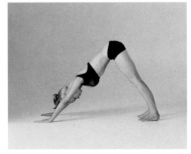 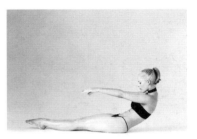

the shoulder bridge series, p121   the leg circles, p67   the up-stretch, p157   >   the leg pull front, p160   >
and the hamstring stretch, p125   >   and the lunge stretch, p69   >

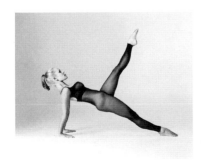 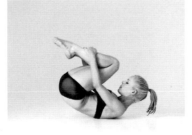 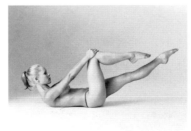 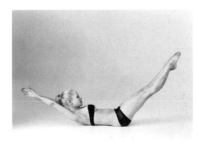

the leg pull back, p163   >   rolling like a ball, p73   >   the single-leg stretch, p74   >   the double-leg stretch, p76   >

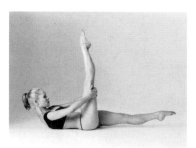

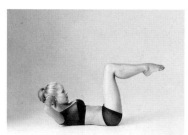

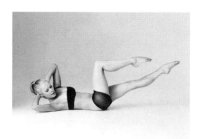

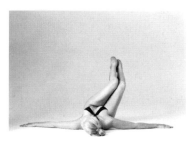

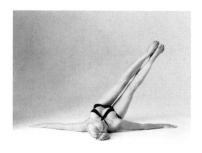

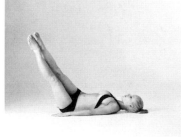

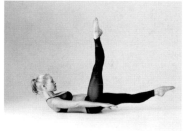

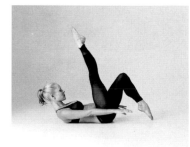

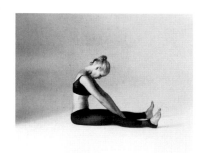

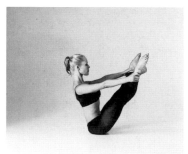

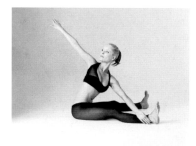

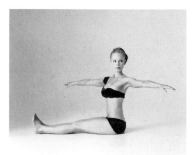

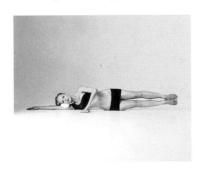

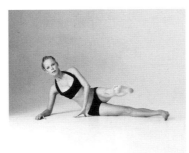

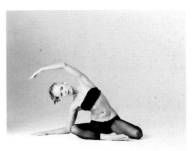

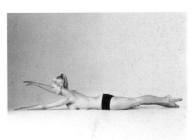

the side lifts, p133
and the quad stretch, p135   >

the side kick i, p137   >

the side bend, p169   >

the mermaid, p176   >

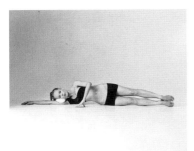

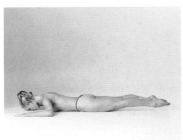

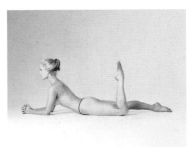

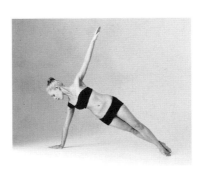

the leg lifts, p141
and the buttock stretch, p143   >

the swan dive, p101   >

the single-leg kick, p104   >

swimming, p154   >

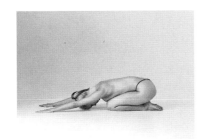

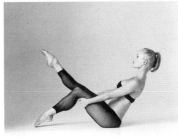

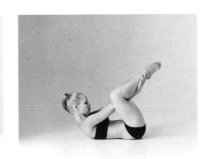

the rest position, p108   >

the teaser prep i & ii, p145   >

the seal puppy, p183

ADVANCED I

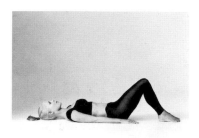

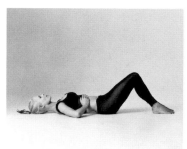

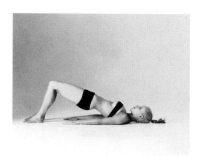

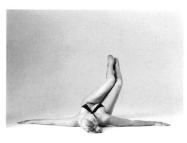

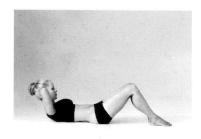

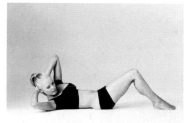

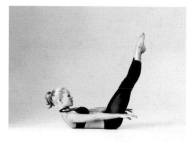

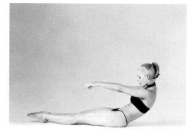

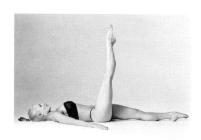

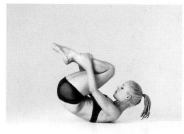

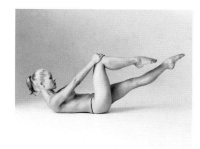

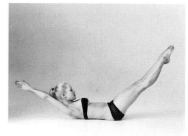

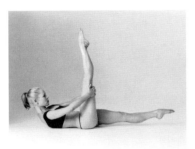 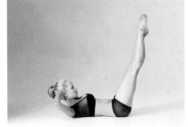 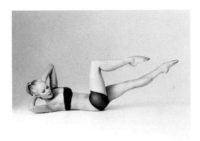 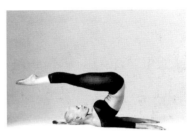

the hamstring pull, p78   >   the double-leg lowers, p80   >   the single-leg stretch twist, p82   >   the roll-over, p63   >

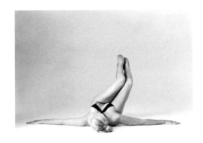 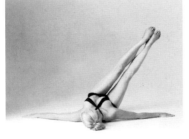 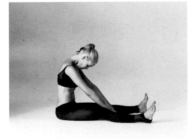 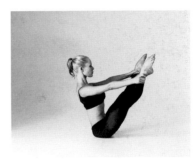

the side to side, p44   >   the pendulum, p92   >   the spine stretch, p85   >   the open-leg rocker, p89   >

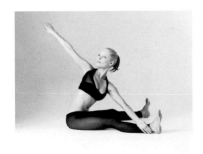 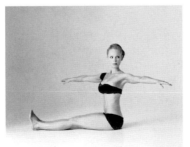 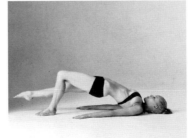 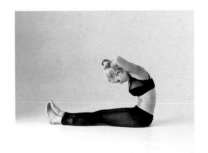

the saw, p98   >   the spine twist, p127   the shoulder bridge series, p121   >   the neck pull, p110   >
and the spine twist stretch, p129   >

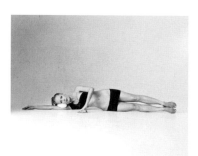

the side lifts, p133
and the quad stretch, p135 >

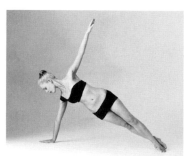

the side bend, p169 >

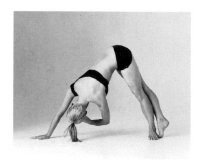

the twist, p173 >

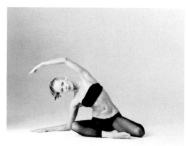

the mermaid, p176 >

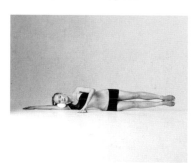

the leg lifts, p141
and the buttock stretch, p143 >

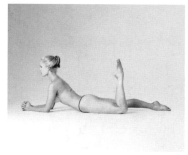

the single-leg kick, p104 >

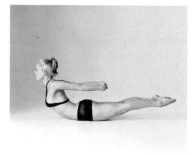

the double-leg kick, p106 >

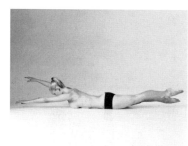

swimming, p154 >

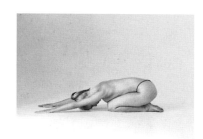

the rest position, p108 >

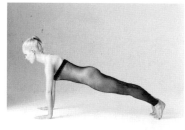

the push-up, p192 >

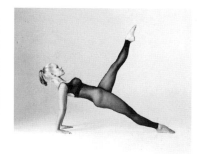

the leg pull back, p163 >

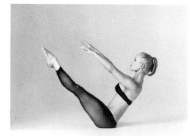

the teaser i, p145 >

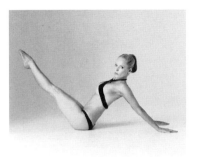

hip circles, p150   >

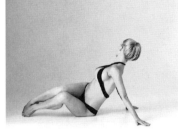

the cancan, p152   >

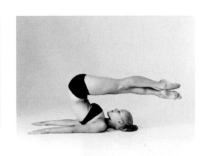

the boomerang, p179

ADVANCED II

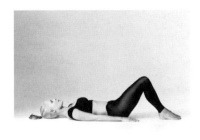

the neutral pelvis & neutral spine, p36   >

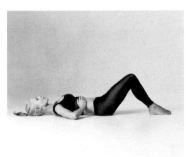

breathing, p38   >

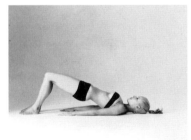

the pelvic roll-up, p41   >

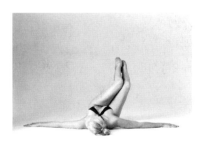

the side to side, p44   >

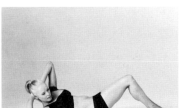

preparation for abdominals, p46   >

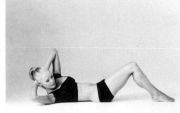

preparation for the twist, p48   >

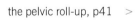

the hundreds, p57   >

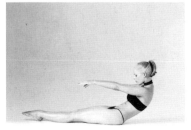

the roll-up, p59   >

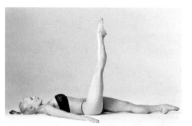

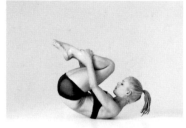

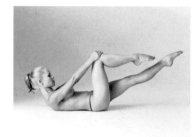

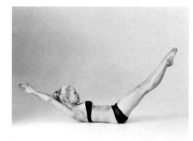

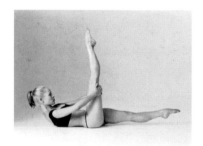

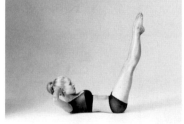

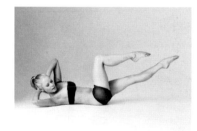

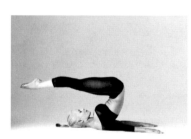

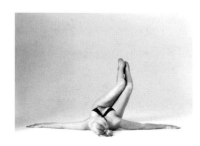

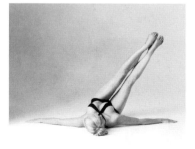

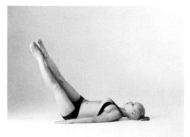

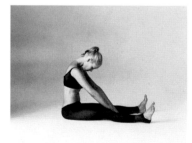

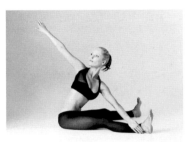

the open-leg rocker, p89 >

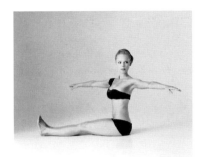

the saw, p98 >

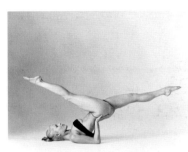

the spine twist, p127 >
and the spine twist stretch, p129 >

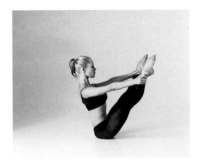

the scissors, p113 >

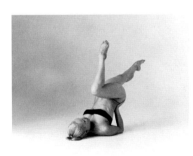

the bicycle, p117 >

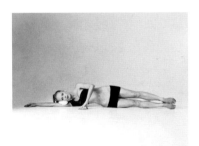

the side lifts, p133
and the quad stretch, p135 >

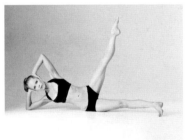

the side kick i, ii & v, p137 >

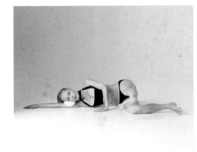

the leg lifts, p141
and the buttock stretch, p143 >

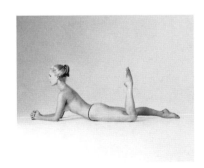

the single-leg kick, p104 >

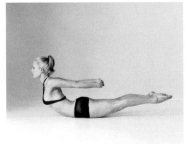

the double-leg kick, p106 >

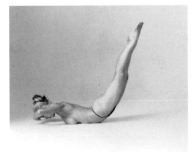

the swan dive, p101 >

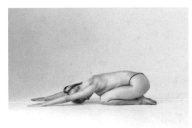

the rest position, p108 >

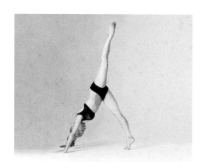

the up-stretch, p157 >

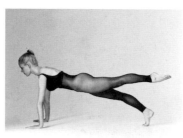

the leg pull front, p160 >

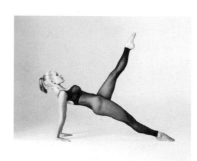

the leg pull back, p163 >

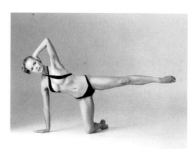

the side kick kneeling, p166 >

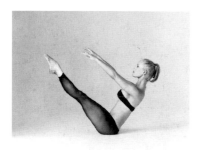

the teaser i, ii & iii, p145 >

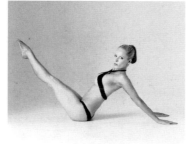

hip circles, p150 >

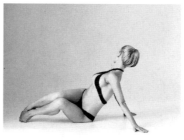

the cancan, p152 >

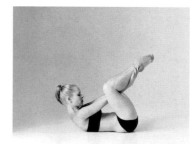

the seal puppy, p183

SUPER-ADVANCED I

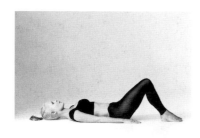

the neutral pelvis & neutral spine,
p36 >

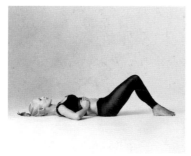

breathing, p38 >

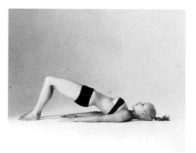

the pelvic roll-up, p41 >

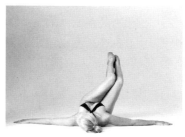

the side to side, p44 >

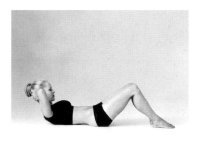

preparation for abdominals, p46 >

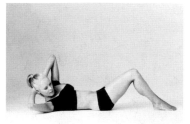

preparation for the twist, p48 >

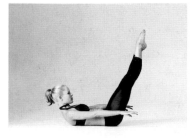

the hundreds, p57 >

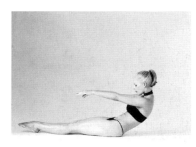

the roll-up, p59 >

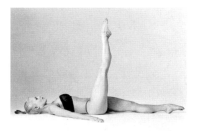

the leg circles, p67 >

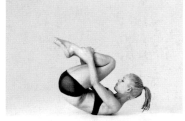

rolling like a ball, p73 >

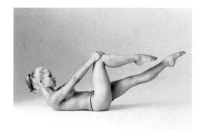

the single-leg stretch, p74 >

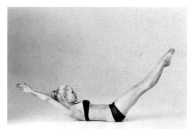

the double-leg stretch, p76 >

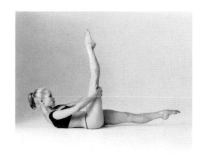

the hamstring pull, p78 >

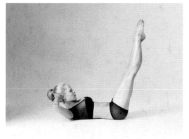

the double-leg lowers, p80 >

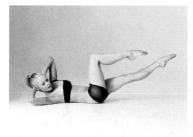

the single-leg stretch twist, p82 >

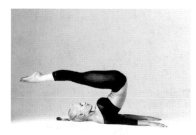

the roll-over, p63 >

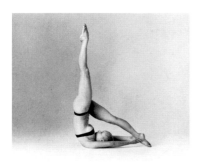

the control balance, p190   >

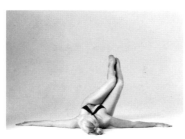

the side to side, p44   >

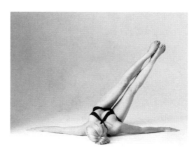

the pendulum, p92   >

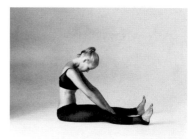

the spine stretch, p85   >

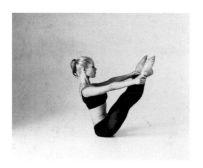

the open-leg rocker, p89   >

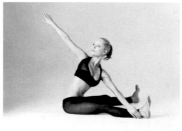

the saw, p98   >

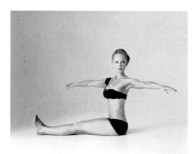

the spine twist, p127   >

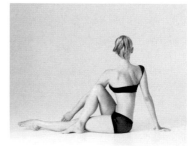

the spine twist stretch, p129   >

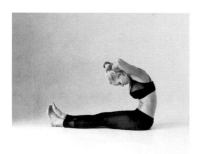

the neck pull, p110   >

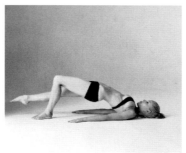

the shoulder bridge series, p121   >

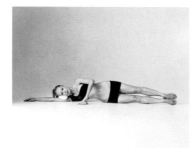

the side lifts, p133
and the quad stretch, p135   >

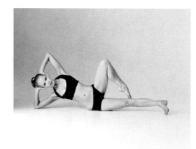

the side kick i, iii & iv, p137   >

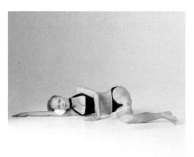

the leg lifts, p141
and the buttock stretch, p143   >

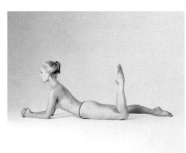

the single-leg kick, p104   >

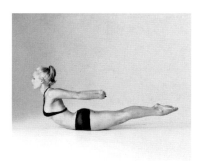

the double-leg kick, p106   >

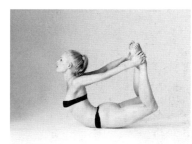

the rocking, p188   >

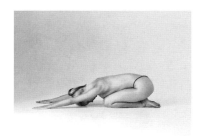

the rest position, p108   >

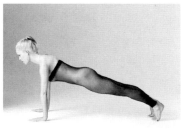

the push-up, p192   >

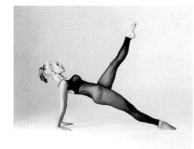

the leg pull back, p163   >

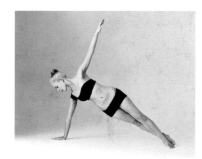

the side bend, p169   >

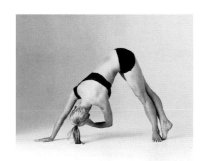

the twist, p173   >

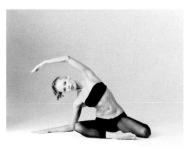

the mermaid, p176   >

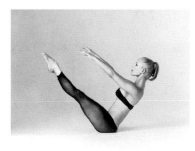

the teaser i, p145   >

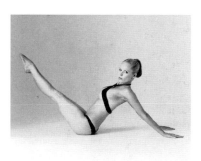

the hip circles, p150   >

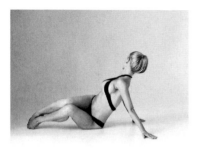

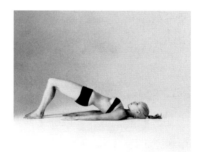

SUPER-ADVANCED II

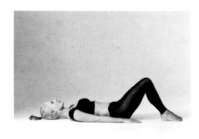

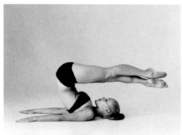

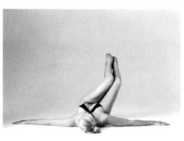

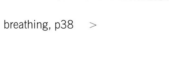

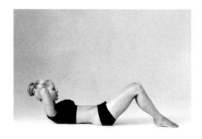

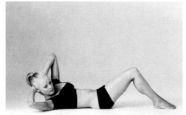

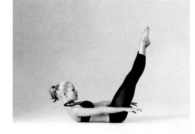

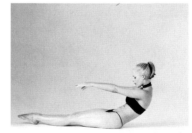

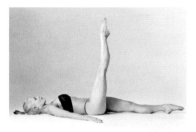

the leg circles, p67 >

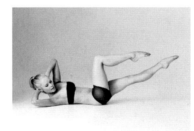

rolling like a ball, p73 >

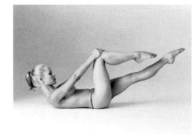

the single-leg stretch, p74 >

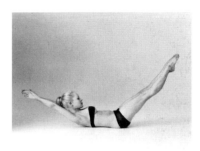

the double-leg stretch, p76 >

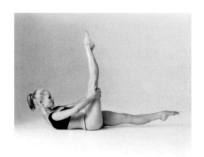

the hamstring pull, p78 >

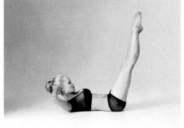

the double-leg lowers, p80 >

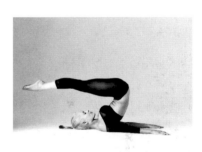

the single-leg stretch twist, p82 >

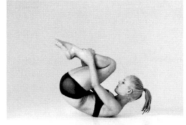

the roll-over, p63 >

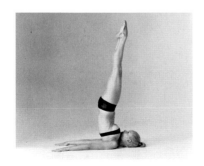

the jackknife, p130 >

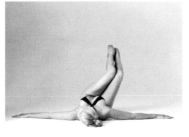

the side to side, p44 >

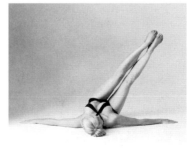

the pendulum, p92 >

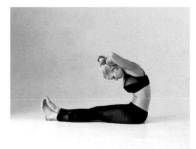

the neck pull, p110 >

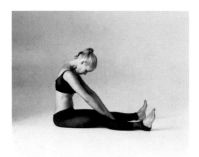

the spine stretch, p85   >

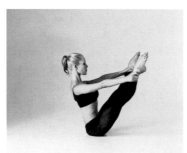

the open-leg rocker, p89   >

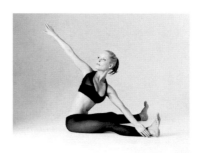

the saw, p98   >

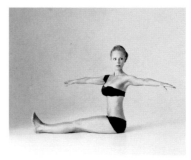

the spine twist, p127   >

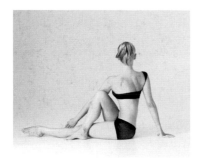

the spine twist stretch, p129   >

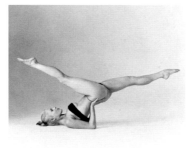

the scissors, p113   >

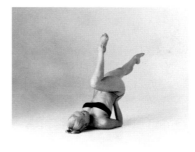

the bicycle, p117   >

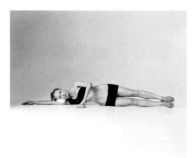

the side lifts, p133
and the quad stretch, p135   >

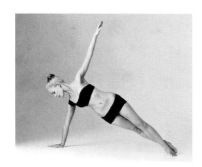

the side bend, p169   >

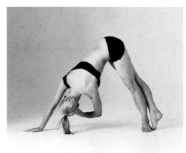

the twist, p173   >

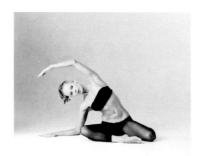

the mermaid, p176   >

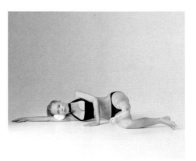

the leg lifts, p141
and the buttock stretch, p143   >

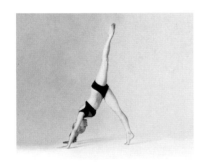

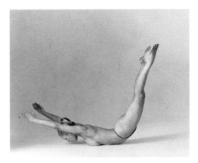

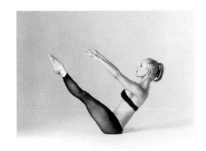

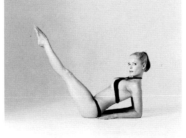

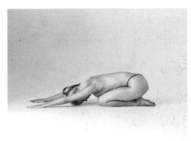

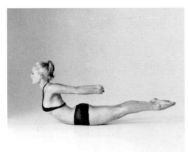

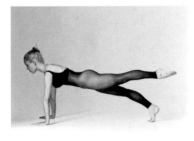

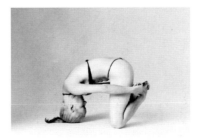

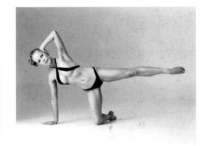

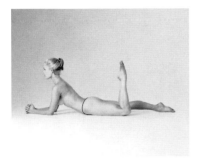

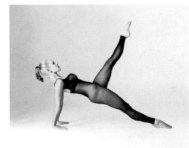

the single-leg kick, p104 >

the double-leg kick, p106 >

the swan dive, p101 >

the rest position, p108 >

the up-stretch, p157 >

the leg pull front, p160 >

the leg pull back, p163 >

the side kick kneeling, p166 >

the teaser i, ii & iii, p145 >

the cancan, p152 >

the crab, p186

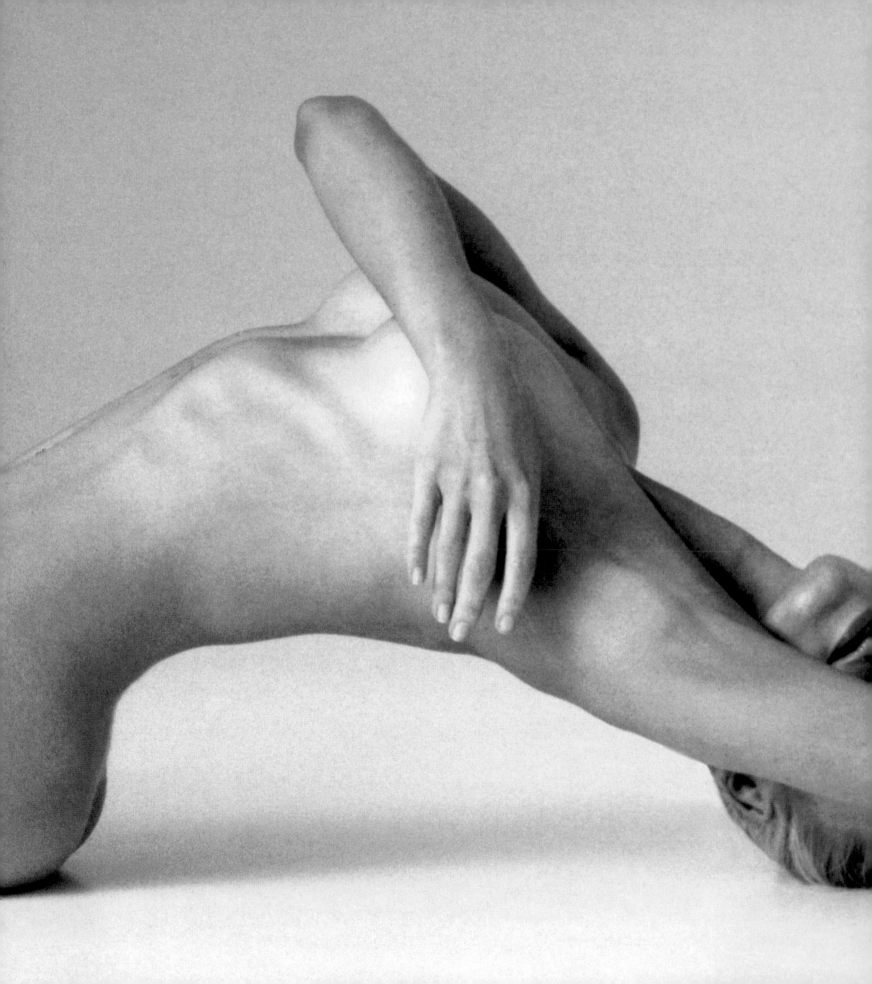

the warm-up

the neutral pelvis & neutral spine

THE NEUTRAL PELVIS

focus Establishing your neutral pelvis.

imagery Visualise a spirit level lying across your pelvis, with the little bubble centred and balanced.

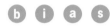

Lie on your back, with your arms relaxed by your sides. Keeping your feet flat on the floor and slightly apart, bend your legs up to a 90-degree angle at the knee joint, and make sure your ankles, knees and hips are in one line.

Visualise each vertebra of your spine melting down into the floor, and focus your awareness on your pelvis.

Breathing naturally, gently rock your pelvis forward and backward, arching and tucking, warming up your lower-back muscles. Notice the distinct difference between the two extremes of movement.

Repetitions: Five sets.

Relax and allow your pelvis to settle into a position between the arch and the tuck. The front of your hip bones and your pubic bone should now all be lying on the same plane. Visualise a glass of water balancing in the centre of your pelvis. This is your neutral pelvis. ①

THE NEUTRAL SPINE

focus Establishing your neutral spine.

imagery Visualise the natural undulations of your spine when you are in a standing position.

tip We each have a unique and beautiful body; your neutral spine will reflect its own individual curves.

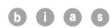

Lie on your back, with your arms relaxed by your sides. Keeping your feet flat on the floor and slightly apart, bend your legs up to a 90-degree angle at the knee joint, and make sure your ankles, knees and hips are in one line.

Focus your awareness on your spine. Notice how your tailbone is gently resting on the floor and feel the natural curve in your lower back. Continuing the journey, feel your ribcage relaxed and gently resting on the floor, feel the natural curve in your neck and feel the back of your head gently resting on the floor. Soften your chin towards your throat, lengthening through the back of your neck. This is your neutral spine. ①

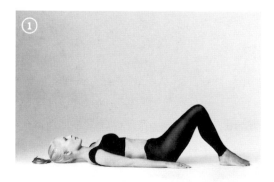

①

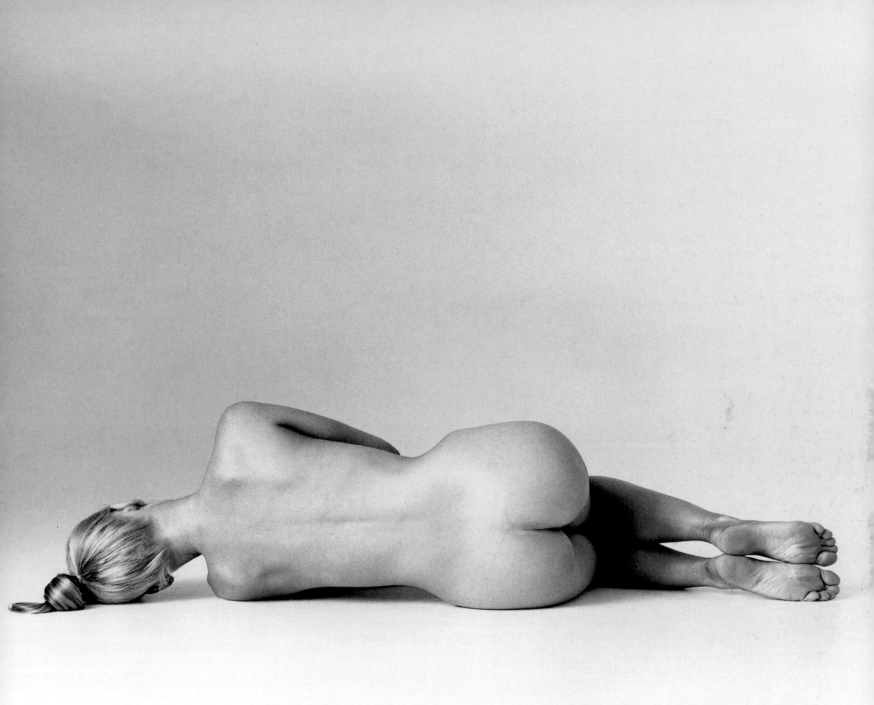

Even in times of quiet repose our body is our source of strength and support.

breathing

BREATHING I

focus Magnifying the way you breathe naturally to create more awareness of your body's subconscious rhythm in daily life.

imagery The natural rise and fall in a baby's tiny body as it breathes.

tip Your deep abdominals have the same nerve supply as your pelvic floor muscles. This means that by firmly engaging either you will work both simultaneously.

Lie on your back, with your hands on the sides of your ribs and your elbows out to your sides. Keeping your feet flat on the floor and together, bend your legs up to a 90-degree angle at the knee joint, and make sure your ankles, knees and hips are in one line. ①

Focus your awareness on your breathing. Breathe in deeply through your nose to the back of your lungs, the sides of your ribs and your abdominals.

Breathe out through your mouth, feeling the natural drop of your ribs and abdominals underneath your hands.

Repetitions: Three.

Move on to Breathing II.

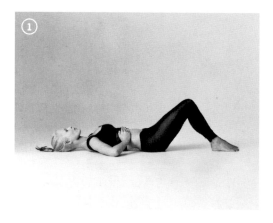

BREATHING II

focus A transition between natural breathing and Pilates breathing.

imagery Visualise drawing your navel towards your spine and spiralling your pelvic floor muscles up towards your ribs.

Continuing on from Breathing I, take a deep breath in through your nose to the back of your lungs, the sides of your ribs and your abdominals. ①

As you breathe out through your mouth, allow your ribs to drop down, draw your navel down towards your spine, tighten your abdominals and lift your pelvic floor muscles, maintaining your neutral pelvis.

Repetitions: Three.

Move on to Breathing III.

BREATHING III

focus Pilates breathing.

imagery Visualise trying to do up the top button of those too-small-for-you jeans that are hiding in the back of your wardrobe!

Continuing on from Breathing II, take a deep breath in through your nose to the back of your lungs and the sides of your ribs, keeping your navel towards your spine. ①

Holding your navel to your spine and keeping your pelvic floor muscles engaged, breathe out through your mouth, drawing your ribs towards your hips.

Repetitions: Three.

This is the style of breathing I would like you to focus on for the rest of your workout.

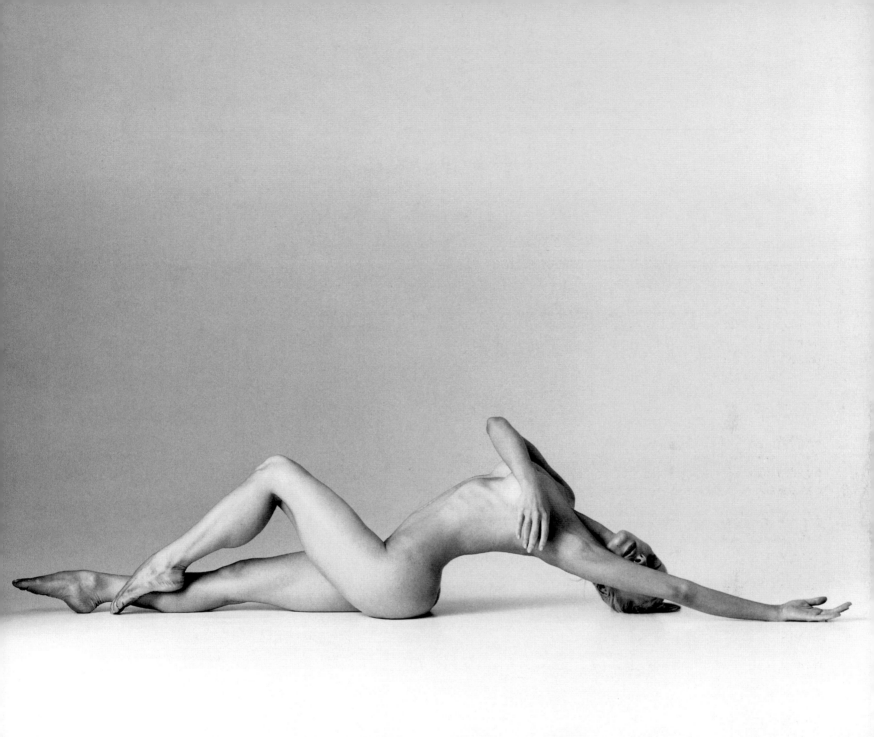

Open your heart and luxuriate in each breath you take, because in breathing we sustain our life force.

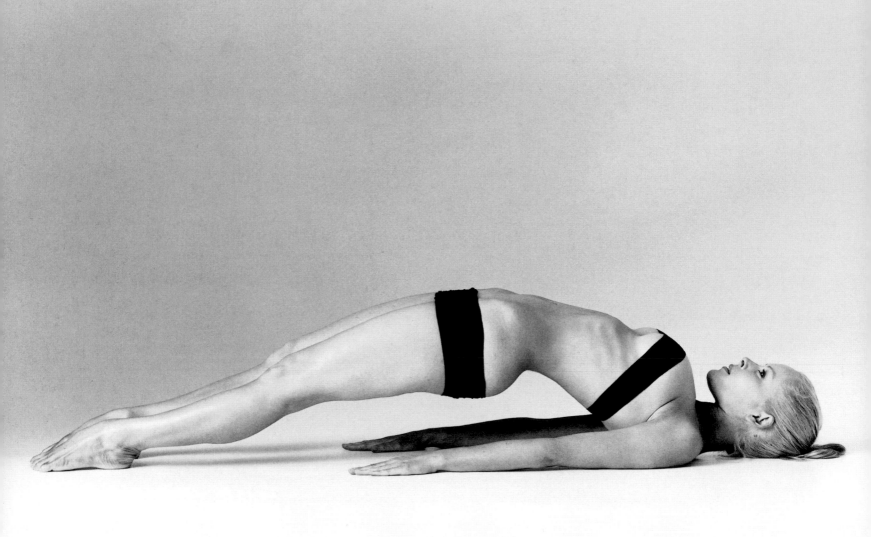

Arching our spine is associated with the sun rising over the horizon; our mind and body awaken with new and expansive vitality.

the pelvic roll-up

focus Spinal articulation and flexibility.

imagery Visualise each vertebra peeling off the floor one at a time smoothly and gracefully.

precaution If you feel any discomfort in your lower back, reduce your movement and return to the start position. Slowly build up your range of movement as you grow stronger.

Lie on your back in the neutral-spine position, with your arms relaxed by your sides. Keeping your feet flat on the floor and slightly apart, bend your legs up to a 90-degree angle at the knee joint, and make sure your ankles, knees and hips are in one line. Draw your navel down towards your spine and tighten your abdominals.

Breathe in to prepare.

As you breathe out, use your abdominals to press your lower back gently onto the floor and lift your tailbone into the air. ① Roll each vertebra up off the floor one at a time and finish with one long, diagonal line between your knees, hips and shoulders. ②

Breathe in and hold the position, maintaining a long neck, with your chin softly held in place.

As you breathe out, starting from your chest slowly lower each vertebra down to the floor one by one, like a string of pearls descending, finishing in the start (neutral-spine) position.

Repetitions: Three.

»

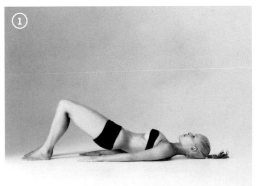

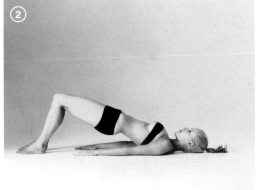

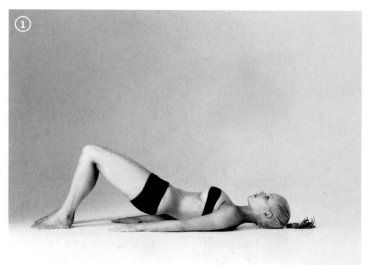

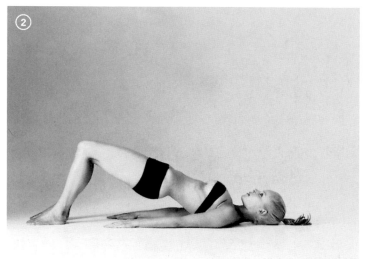

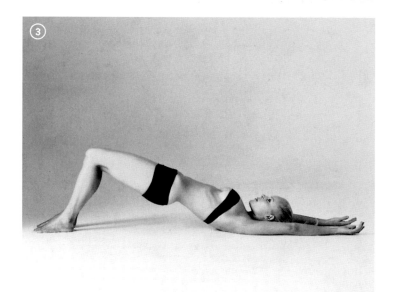

THE PELVIC ROLL-UP WITH ARM CIRCLES

focus Spinal articulation and shoulder mobilisation.

imagery Visualise each vertebra peeling off the floor one at a time smoothly and gracefully.

precaution If you feel any discomfort in your lower back or shoulders, reduce your movement and return to the start position. Slowly build up your range of movement as you grow stronger.

Lie on your back in the neutral-spine position, with your arms relaxed by your sides. Keeping your feet flat on the floor and slightly apart, bend your legs up to a 90-degree angle at the knee joint, and make sure your ankles, knees and hips are in one line. Draw your navel down towards your spine and tighten your abdominals.

Breathe in to prepare.

As you breathe out, use your abdominals to press your lower back gently onto the floor and lift your tailbone into the air. ① Roll each vertebra up off the floor one at a time and finish with one long, diagonal line between your knees, hips and shoulders. ②

As you breathe in, reach both arms up towards the ceiling and allow them to float back onto the floor behind you. ③

As you breathe out, starting from your chest slowly lower each vertebra down to the floor one by one, like a string of pearls descending, finishing in the start (neutral-spine) position, your shoulders and arms relaxed and still.

As you breathe in, sweep your arms around your sides along the floor and back to their start position.

Repetitions: Three.

the side to side

focus Rotation and the sides of your abdominals.

imagery Visualise your chest as a lead weight enabling you to move only the lower half of your body freely into an effective stretch.

precaution If you feel any discomfort in your lower back, place your feet together on the floor and reduce your movement to a pain-free zone.

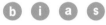

Lie on your back, with your knees lifted in a tabletop position (90 degrees at hip and knee) and squeezed together. Stretch your arms out to your sides, aligned with your chest, with your palms face-down. Anchor your tailbone and use your abdominals and the back of your ribs to keep your spine flat on the floor. ①

Breathe in to prepare, keeping your knees squeezed together and on the same plane.

As you breathe out, roll your head to the left as you carry both knees over to the right, allowing your hips, waist and ribs to follow gracefully. Keep your knees on the same plane and your left shoulder and shoulder blade firmly planted on the floor, indulging

in the stretch behind your ribcage and at the front of your chest. ②

As you breathe in, initiating from your abdominals draw your ribs, waist, hips and knees back to the start position, and roll your head back to the centre.

Repetitions: Three alternating to each side.

THE THORACO LUMBAR STRETCH

focus To release tension in the area between your ribs and pelvis. This stretch can be used in conjunction with any exercise that involves rotation, to increase your range of movement.

precaution Stop if you feel any lower-back discomfort during the stretch.

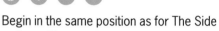

Begin in the same position as for The Side to Side. ①

Carry both knees over to the left, allowing your legs to relax onto the floor. Try to keep your right shoulder firmly planted on the floor like a lead weight, and place your left arm over your thighs and knees to anchor your position. Hold this position for six full, deep breaths before changing to the other side. ③

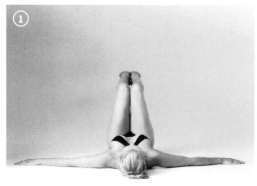

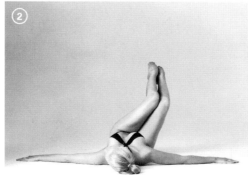

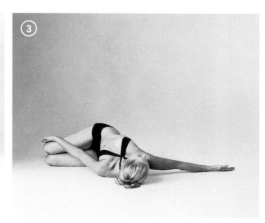

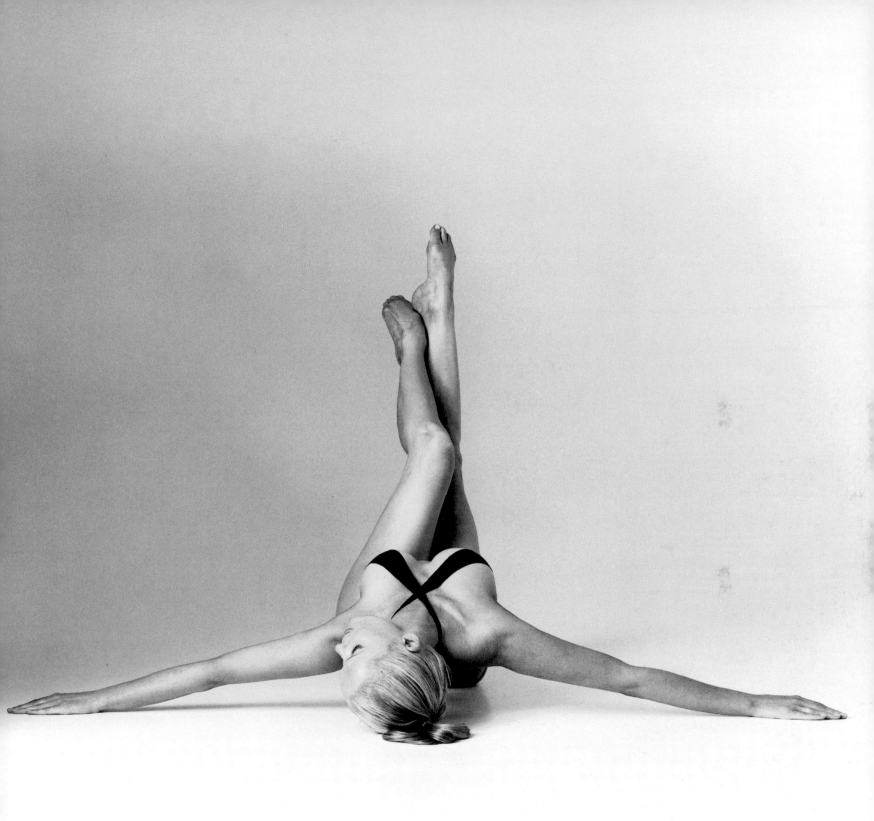

Indulge your body for a moment in the simple beauty of movement.

preparation for abdominals

focus Spinal flexion and abdominals.

imagery Think of a piece of string running from your tailbone to the crown of your head, lengthening your spine.

tip For maximum benefit, keep your tailbone down, curl forward to an angle of 30 degrees and keep the front of your hips soft.

b **i** **a** **s**

Lie on your back, with your spine in neutral. Keeping your feet flat on the floor and slightly apart, bend your legs up to a 90-degree angle at the knee joint, and make sure your ankles, knees and hips are in one line. Place your hands behind your head and link your fingers together, with your thumbs working down the back of your neck. Draw your navel firmly towards your spine and lift your pelvic floor muscles.

Breathe in as you gently pull on your neck, stretching the crown of your head to the wall behind you and creating a pocket of space between each vertebra.

Keeping your tailbone anchored and your head heavily in your hands, breathe out as you curl your head, neck and chest forward, drawing your ribs towards your hips.
Keep your eye-line focused on the top of your kneecaps.

Hold the position as you breathe in to the back of your lungs and the sides of your ribs, keeping your abdominals firm and your tailbone anchored.

Breathe out as you slowly roll your spine back down to the floor.

Repetitions: Three.

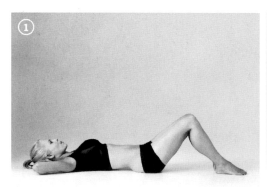
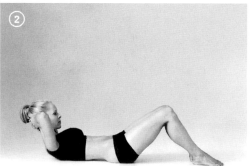

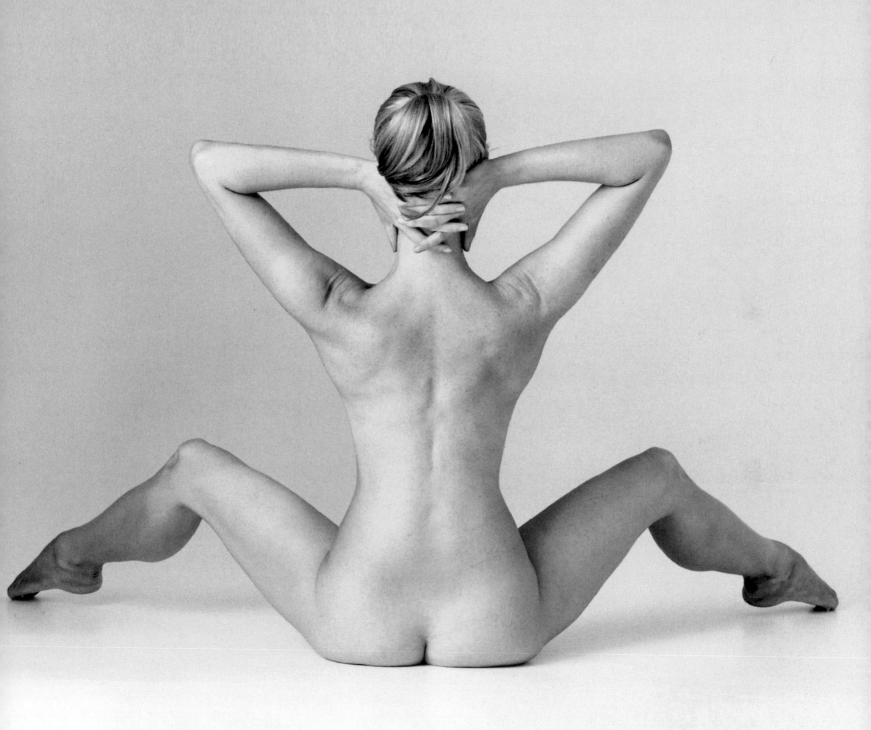

Balance and alignment are the foundations of beautiful posture.

preparation for the twist

focus The sides of your abdominals, spinal flexion and rotation.

imagery Think of a piece of string running from your tailbone to the crown of your head, lengthening the back of your spine.

Lie on your back, with your spine in neutral. Keeping your feet flat on the floor and slightly apart, bend your legs up to a 90-degree angle at the knee joint, and make sure your ankles, knees and hips are in one line. Place your hands behind your head and link your fingers together, with your thumbs working down the back of your neck. Draw your navel firmly towards your spine. ①

Breathe in as you gently pull on your neck, stretching the crown of your head back towards the wall and creating a pocket of space between each vertebra.

As you breathe out, curl your chest forward and take your left shoulder towards your right knee, keeping your elbows open, your hips and knees still and your tailbone anchored. ②

As you breathe in to the back of your lungs and the sides of your ribs, return your upper body to centre, keeping your chest high and your abdominals firm. ③

As you breathe out, take your right shoulder towards your left knee, keeping your elbows open, your hips and knees still and your tailbone anchored.

As you breathe in, return to centre, keeping your chest high and your tailbone anchored.

Repetitions: Three alternating each way.

Finish the last repetition with your head and chest lifted in the centre position.

Breathe out as you roll your chest, neck and head back down to the floor, vertebra by vertebra, finishing in the neutral-spine position.

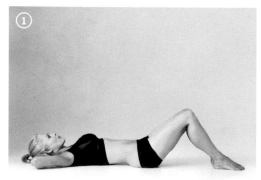

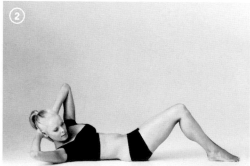

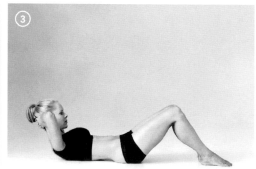

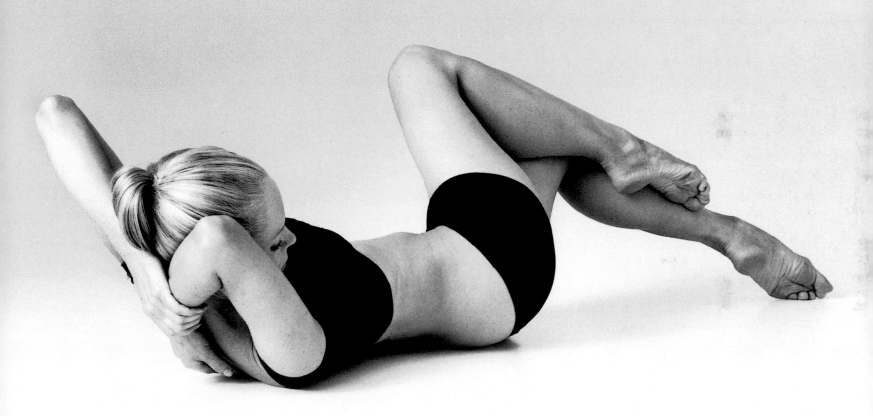

As your body becomes more in tune with your mind, take a moment to discover your inner self. Awakening your intuition is the first step in understanding your body's untapped potential.

preparation for the hundreds

focus Abdominals and flowing movement.

precaution If you feel any discomfort in your lower back, keep your toes in contact with the floor throughout the exercise. If you have any discomfort in your shoulders, reduce the range of your arm movement to a pain-free zone.

b **i**

Lie on your back, with your spine in neutral, your legs stretched out flat along the floor and your inner thighs squeezed together. Stretch your arms out on the floor behind you and draw your navel firmly towards your spine. Sink the back of your ribcage down into the floor and relax your shoulders. Point your toes. ①

Breathe in as you bend your legs, sliding your toes along the floor until your knees are at a 90-degree angle, keeping your spine neutral, your abdominals firm and the back of your ribs anchored. ②

Keeping your tailbone anchored, breathe out as you curl forward, lifting your chest, bringing your arms over your head towards your hips and stretching your legs straight up into the air. ③

Keeping your chest lifted, breathe in and bend your legs at the knees, touching your toes back onto the floor. ④

Breathe out as you return to the start position, sliding your toes along the floor as you reach your arms over your head and back onto the floor behind you.

Repetitions: Five.

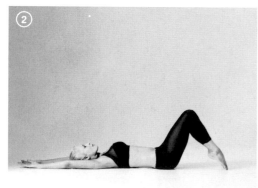

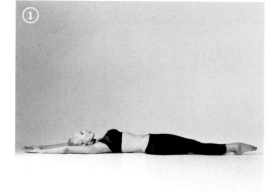

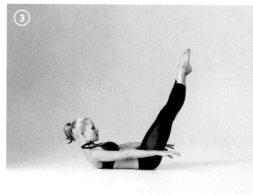

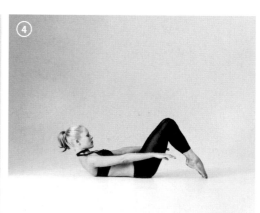

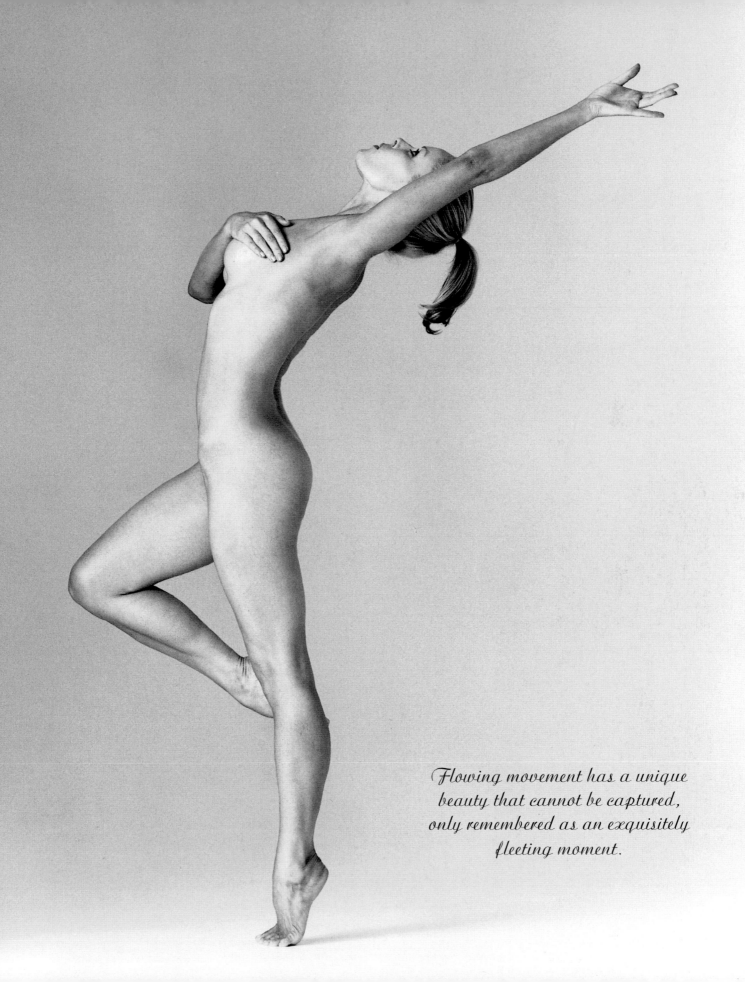

Flowing movement has a unique beauty that cannot be captured, only remembered as an exquisitely fleeting moment.

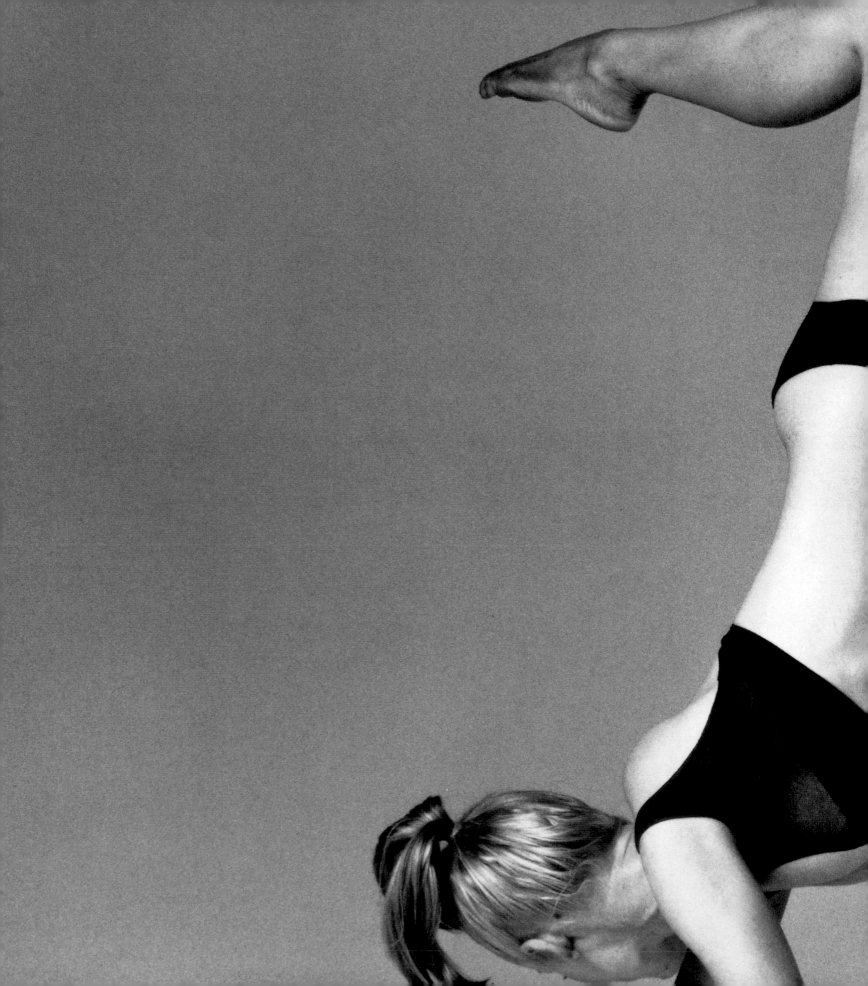

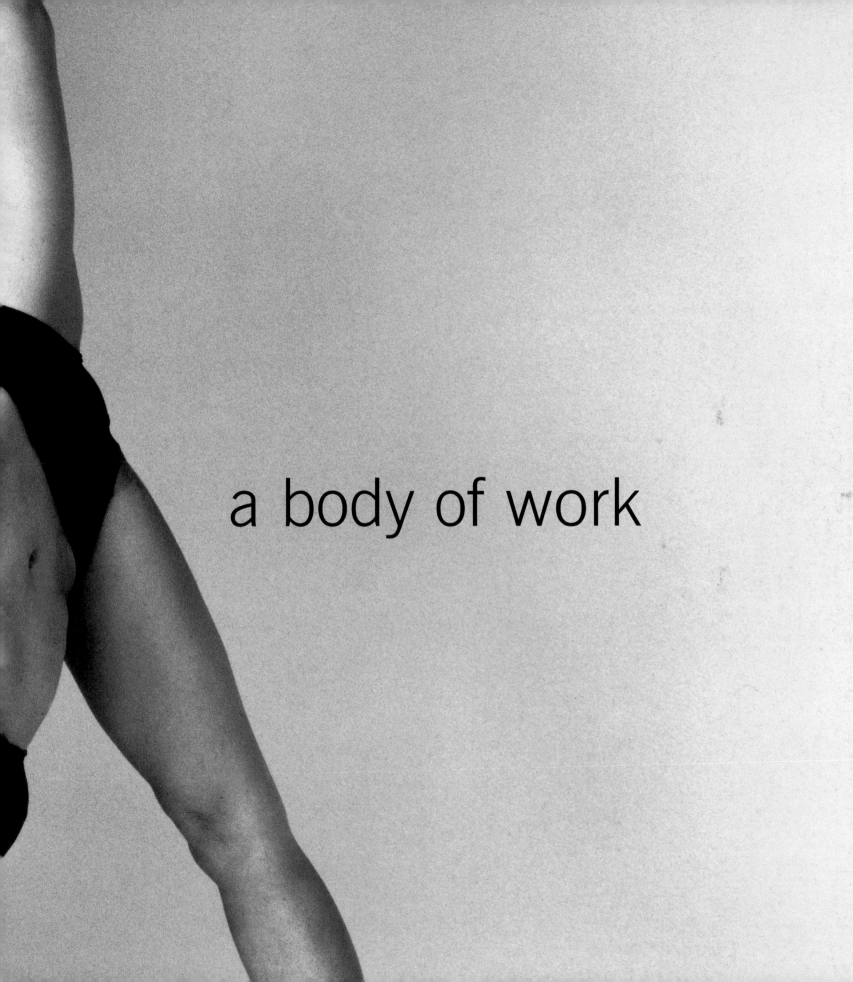

a body of work

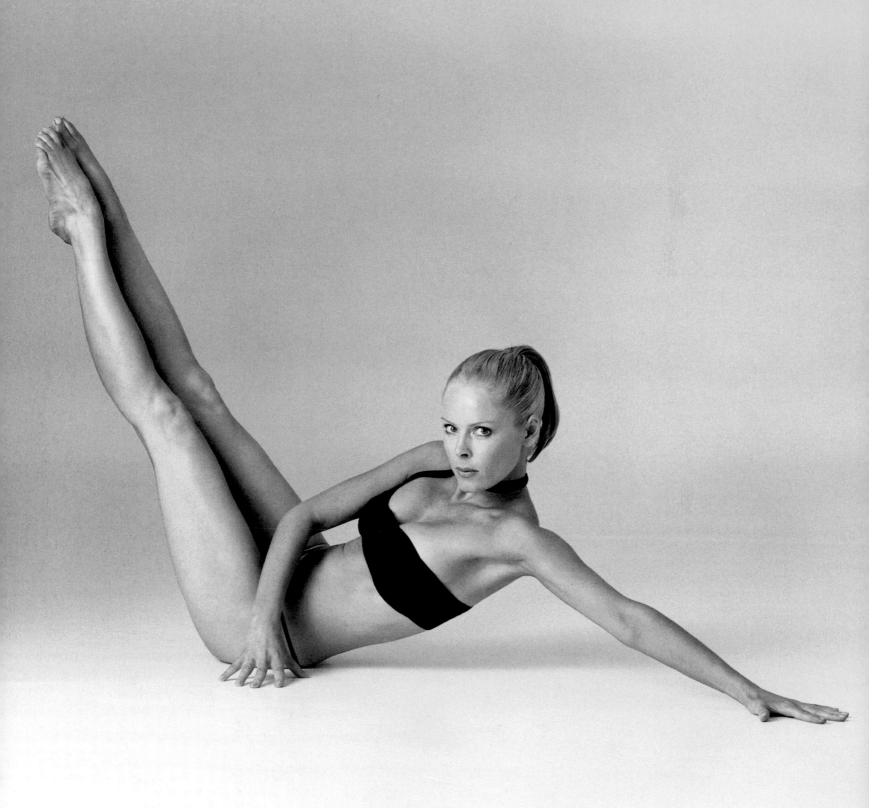

Some of the most challenging experiences in life are masked within what appears to be a simple exterior.

the hundreds

ESTABLISHING YOUR HUNDREDS POSITION

tip Your Hundreds position is unique to your body, so find a position that is comfortable but personally challenging.

Lie on your back, with your spine in neutral, your legs stretched out flat along the floor and your inner thighs squeezed together. Stretch your arms out on the floor behind you and draw your navel firmly towards your spine. Sink the back of your ribcage down into the floor and relax your shoulders. Point your toes. ①

Breathe in and bend your legs, sliding your toes along the floor until your knees are at a 90-degree angle, keeping your spine neutral, your abdominals firm and the back of your ribs anchored. ②

Keeping your tailbone anchored, breathe out as you curl forward, lifting your chest, bringing your arms over your head towards your hips and stretching your legs straight up into the air. ③

Place your hands behind your head and link your fingers together, with your thumbs working down the back of your neck, and practise your

Pilates breathing (breathing in and out through the back of your lungs and the sides of your ribs, keeping your abdominals and pelvic floor muscles firm, see page 38).

From this position you need to establish your ideal leg alignment to challenge your abdominals and maintain a relaxed and safe lower back.

If you feel any tightness or weakness in your lower back, bend your legs at the knees until your focus is back on your abdominals (this makes the exercise easier).

To make the exercise harder, keep your legs straight and lower them to a safe but challenging angle.

Whichever position feels strong in your abdominals and safe in your lower back is your Hundreds position.

»

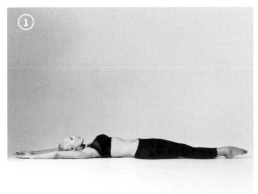

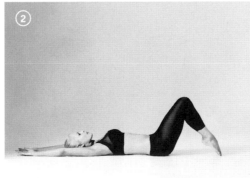

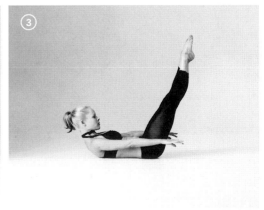

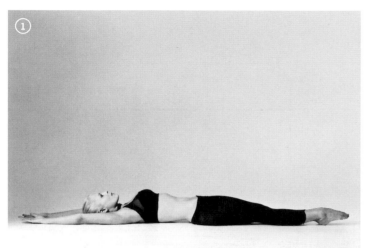

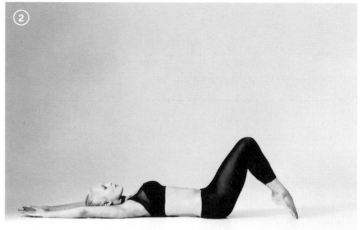

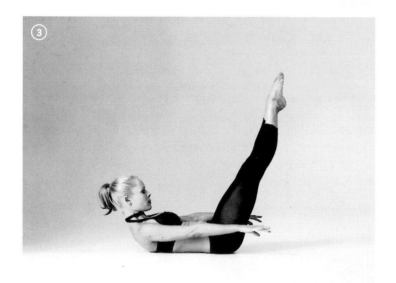

THE HUNDREDS

focus Shoulder girdle stability, abdominals and endurance.

precaution Stop if you feel any lower-back discomfort. Remember that one of the focus points is endurance, so build yourself up gradually. If you feel any discomfort in the back of your neck, support your head with your hands throughout the exercise.

point of interest The Hundreds exercise is considered the signature exercise of the Pilates Method. If you haven't done The Hundreds, you haven't done Pilates!

Lie on your back, with your spine in neutral, your legs stretched out flat along the floor and your inner thighs squeezed together. Stretch your arms out on the floor behind you and draw your navel firmly towards your spine. Sink the back of your ribcage down into the floor and relax your shoulders. Point your toes. ①

Breathe in and bend your legs at the knees, sliding your toes along the floor until your knees are at a 90-degree angle, keeping your spine neutral, your abdominals firm and the back of your ribs anchored. ②

Keeping your tailbone anchored, breathe out as you curl forward into your Hundreds position, lifting your chest, bringing your arms stretched out towards your hips and your legs stretched up into the air. ③

As you breathe in, pump your arms up and down five times with small, strong movements, keeping the back of your arms firm. Focus on maintaining a very still torso, allowing your arms to move independently, dissociating your arms from your shoulders.

As you breathe out, pump your arms up and down five times with small, strong movements.

Repetitions: Ten.

Keeping your chest lifted, breathe in and bend your legs at the knees, touching your toes back onto the floor.

As you breathe out, return to the start position, sliding your toes along the floor as you reach your arms over your head and back onto the floor behind you.

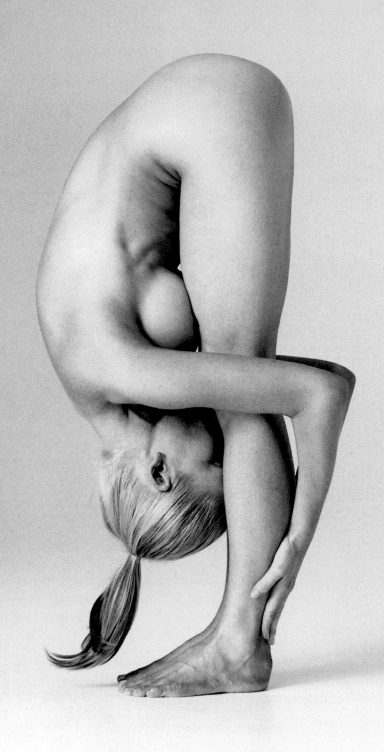

Flexibility in both our mind and body allows us the freedom to explore new horizons.

the roll-up

focus Spinal articulation, and the coordination and integration between the abdominals and hip flexors.

imagery Visualise your spine as a string of pearls peeling off the floor and returning one at a time smoothly and gracefully.

precaution Stop if you feel any discomfort in your lower back.

tip The abdominals are the predominant muscles for the first 30 degrees of spinal flexion; between 30 and 35 degrees there is a transition between the abdominals and the hip flexors; the hip flexors complete the movement. Our bodies have difficulty smoothly making the transition, but with time and patience you will develop the strength to achieve this goal. Allow your body to remain at beginner level until you can smoothly complete the transition.

b

Lie on your back, with your legs in a tabletop position (90 degrees at the hip and knee), your feet flexed and your hands holding onto the back of your thighs.

Breathe in to prepare.

As you breathe out, push the backs of your thighs into your hands as you roll forward, maintaining a C-curve (shoulders over hips and navel curved back behind your pelvis). Point your feet, place them on the floor and slide them out in front of you.

Drape your body over your thighs and stretch out your spine and the backs of your legs, and reach your hands out towards your ankles.

Take hold of your legs, aiming to hold on as closely as possible to your ankles.

Breathe in and hold the stretch.

As you breathe out, draw your chest closer to your thighs, keeping your arms in the same position.

»

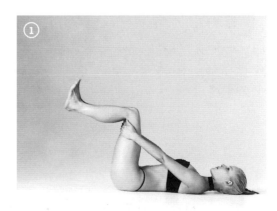

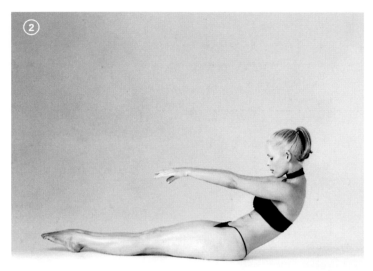

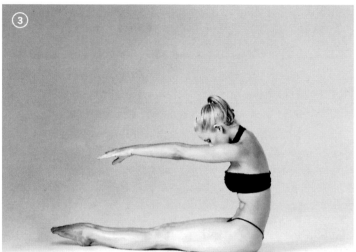

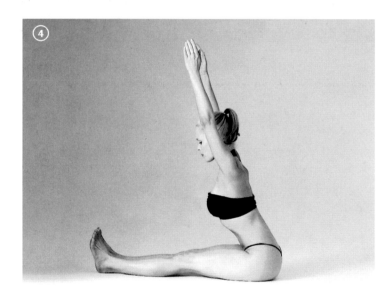

As you breathe in, bend your legs at the knees, sliding your feet along the floor, maintaining a C-curve in your body and your hands once again holding on behind your thighs.

As you breathe out, roll your spine back down onto the floor, pushing into your hands with the back of your thighs, and finishing in the start position.

Repetitions: Six.

Lie on your back, with your legs stretched out flat along the floor, your inner thighs squeezed together and your feet pointed. Stretch your arms out on the floor behind you, draw your navel towards your spine and relax your ribcage and shoulders.

As you breathe in, curl your head and shoulders forward and lift your arms off the floor, passing them over your chest and reaching your fingers towards your toes.

Drawing your navel towards your spine, breathe out as you peel your spine off the floor vertebra by vertebra. ②

Drape your body over your thighs, stretching your spine and the back of your legs, and reach your hands out towards your ankles.

Breathe in and hold the stretch.

As you breathe out, flex your feet and pull yourself down closer to your thighs to increase the stretch.

Breathe in and hold the stretch.

As you breathe out, point your feet and roll your spine back down to the floor, vertebra by vertebra, returning to the start position.

Repetitions: Six.

Lie on your back, with your legs stretched out flat along the floor, your inner thighs squeezed together and your feet pointed. Stretch your arms out on the floor behind you, draw your navel towards your spine and relax your ribcage and shoulders.

As you breathe in, curl your head and shoulders forward and lift your arms off the floor, passing them over your chest and reaching your fingers towards your toes.

As you breathe out, peel your spine off the floor vertebra by vertebra. ② Finish in a C-curve, with your arms parallel to the floor. ③

As you breathe in, straighten your spine and sit tall, and reach both hands out to your sides at chest height, palms face-down.

As you breathe out, lift your arms above your head and lean forward on an incline, with your arms by your ears and your feet flexed. Visualise a long line running from the base of your spine to the tips of your fingers. ④

As you breathe in, return to the C-curve position, with your shoulders down, your chest relaxed and soft, and your feet pointed.

As you breathe out, roll your spine down, vertebra by vertebra, returning to the start position.

Repetitions: Six.

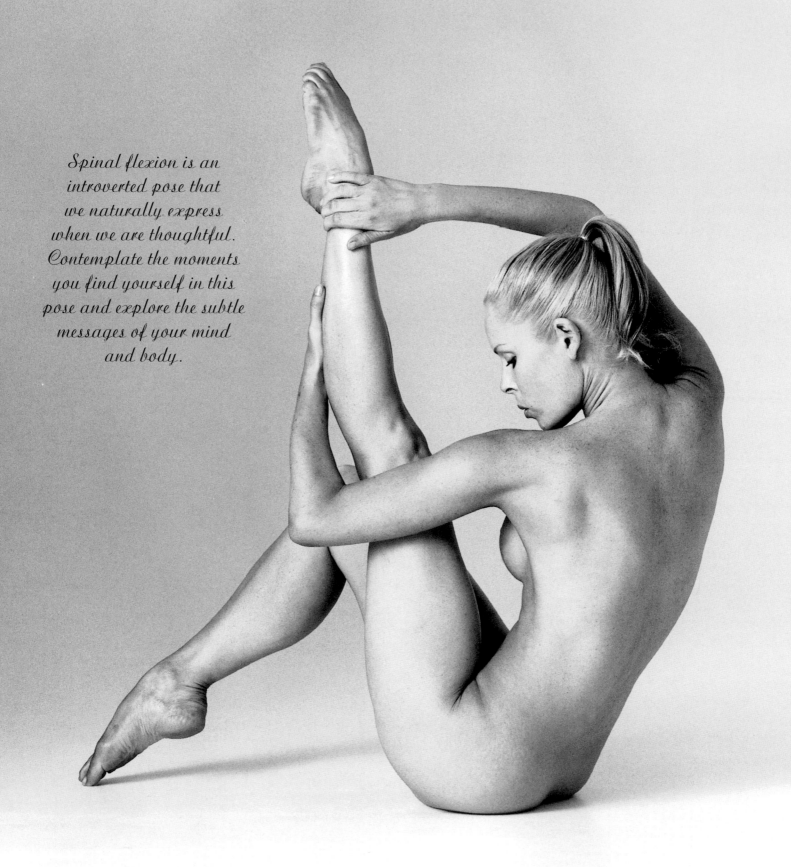

Spinal flexion is an introverted pose that we naturally express when we are thoughtful. Contemplate the moments you find yourself in this pose and explore the subtle messages of your mind and body.

the roll-over

focus Spinal articulation and control.

imagery As you roll over and back, think of hollowing your abdominals out with an ice-cream scoop.

precaution If you have a neck or lower-back issue, obtain clearance from your treating practitioner before attempting this exercise. This exercise should be performed for the first time under experienced supervision.

Lie on your back, with your arms by your sides, your legs lifted straight (90 degrees at the hip) and squeezed together, and your feet pointed. Draw your navel towards your spine, anchoring your tailbone. ①

Breathe in to prepare.

As you breathe out, focus on using your abdominals to carry your legs over your head until they finish parallel to the floor and your body weight is balanced between your shoulder blades. Keep your arms strongly imprinted on the floor beside you. ②

Keeping your legs straight, breathe in as you lower them towards your chest and the floor, flexing your feet.

Maintaining an open chest and keeping your arms firmly imprinted on the floor, breathe out, with your chin slightly tucked, lengthening through the back of your neck. Roll your spine back down to the floor vertebra by vertebra, with your thighs as close to your chest as possible, stretching out your spine and the back of your thighs, finishing in the start position.

Repetitions: Two.

»

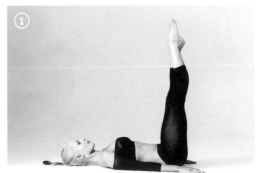

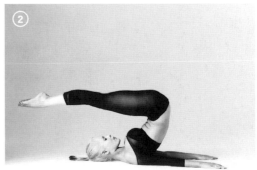

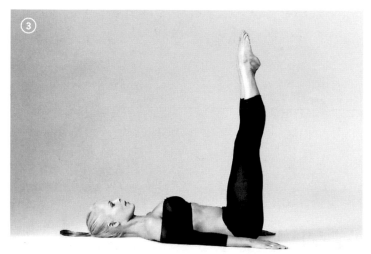

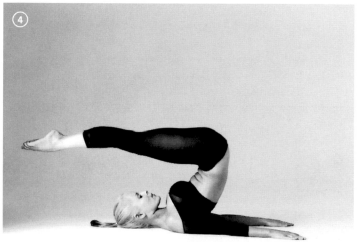

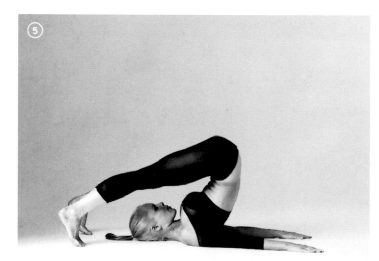

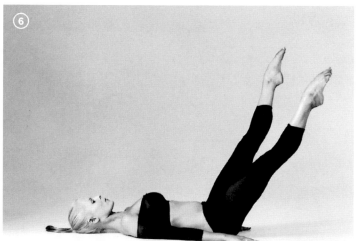

Continuing on, visualise the shape of a long oval; this is the shape you will soon draw with your legs. As you breathe in, hold your legs in the start position. ③

As you breathe out, focus on using your abdominals to carry your legs over your head until they finish parallel to the floor and your body weight is balanced between your shoulder blades. Keep your arms strongly imprinted on the floor beside you. ④

Keeping your legs straight, breathe in as you lower them towards your chest and the floor, flexing and separating your feet until they are shoulder-width apart. ⑤

Maintaining an open chest and keeping your arms firmly imprinted on the floor, breathe out, with your chin slightly tucked, lengthening through the back of your neck and roll your spine back down to the floor vertebra by vertebra, with your thighs as close to your chest as possible, stretching out your spine and the back of your thighs.

As you breathe in, point your feet, squeeze your buttocks and lower your legs forward towards the floor, as far as possible without your pelvis or lower back moving. Draw your inner thighs together and lift your legs back up to the start position, completing an oval shape with your legs. ⑥

Repetitions: Two.

Now reverse your ovals by breathing out as you squeeze your buttocks and lower your legs forward towards the floor, as far as possible without your pelvis or lower back moving, with your inner thighs squeezed together.

Keeping your toes pointed, separate your feet until they are shoulder-width apart. Breathe in as you draw your legs up until you have a 90-degree angle at your hip joint.

As you breathe out, focus on using your abdominals to carry your legs over your head until they finish parallel to the floor and your body weight is balanced between your shoulder blades. Keep your arms strongly imprinted on the floor beside you. ④

Keeping your legs straight, breathe in as you lower them towards your chest and the floor, flexing your feet and squeezing your inner thighs together.

Maintaining an open chest and keeping your arms firmly imprinted on the floor, breathe out, with your chin slightly tucked, lengthening through the back of your neck. Roll your spine back down to the floor vertebra by vertebra, with your thighs as close to your chest as possible, stretching out your spine and the back of your thighs with your feet flexed.

Breathe in as you hold your start position, pointing your feet.

Repetitions: Two.

variation ⓢ

Rather than opening your legs shoulder-width apart, open them as wide as you can, allowing your oval shape to become big circles.

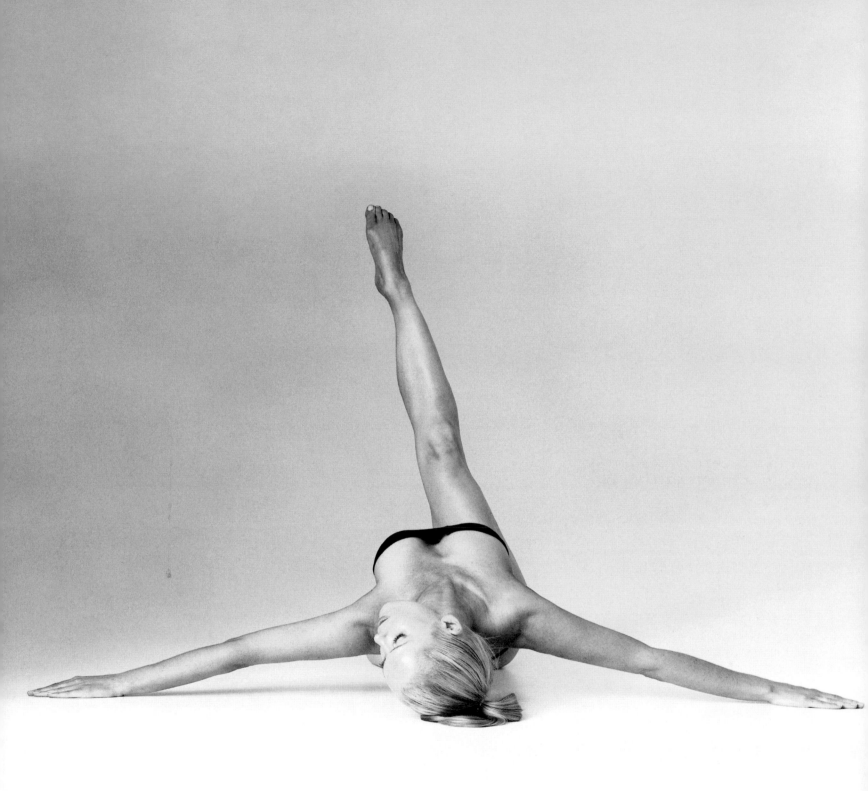

Fluid movement is exhilarating and refreshing. Explore your mental and physical boundaries and then challenge them further with confidence, reaching out to each new and wonderful experience.

the leg circles

focus Pelvic stability and the front of the thighs.

imagery Stirring a pot of thick chicken soup with your leg.

tip This is an intense exercise, and yes, it hurts! Only use the precautions if you really do have the issues mentioned; otherwise, soldier on. Follow this exercise with The Lunge Stretch (see page 69) for the beginner–intermediate variation, which is much slower than the original, in order to teach you impeccable technique. Once you reach the advanced level, your leg circles become faster and less stressful to the front of your thighs, therefore eliminating the need to insert The Lunge Stretch.

Lie on your back, with your spine in neutral, your hands by your sides and your palms face-down. Press the back of your left thigh firmly into the floor, keeping your heel anchored and your foot softly pointed. Stretch your right leg up into the air and hold it straight, with your foot softly pointed. (The height of the lifted leg is different for everyone; ensure you can comfortably maintain a neutral spine. The more flexible you are, the higher you will be able to hold your leg to begin.) Draw your navel firmly towards your spine, narrowing your waist. ①

If you feel any discomfort in your lower back, bend your underneath knee. ② If you have an injury or restriction in your hip flexors, bend

your working leg to a tabletop position (90 degrees at the hip and knee). ③

Breathe in to prepare.

As you breathe out, open your right leg out to the side and circle it down, focusing on using your abdominals and the pressure of the back of your left thigh on the floor to keep your pelvis stable.

As you breathe in, continue the circle, maintaining a stable pelvis, allowing your right leg to pass over your centre line and return to the start position.

Repetitions: Ten in each direction before changing to the other leg.

variation **a**

Follow the steps for the beginner–intermediate level, but complete your first circle while breathing in, then your second circle while breathing out.

Repetitions: Ten in each direction before changing to the other leg.

variation **s**

To challenge yourself even further, complete the advanced variation with both arms straight and reaching above your chest, with your palms facing each other, your shoulders drawing down towards your hips and your chest open. »

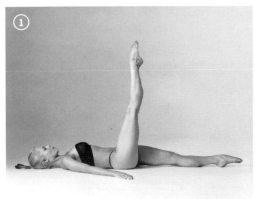

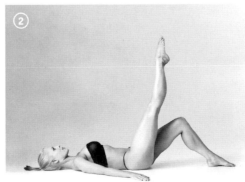

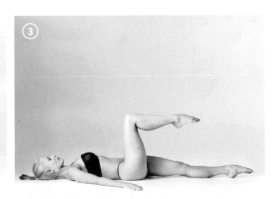

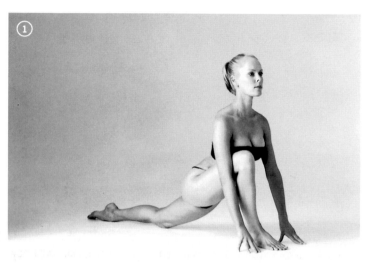
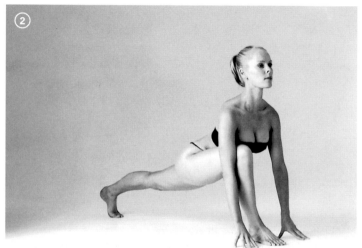

THE LUNGE STRETCH

focus This is a static stretch to lengthen out the hip flexor muscles at the front of your hip, relieving any excess tension created from keeping the beginner–intermediate variation slow and controlled.

precaution If you feel any discomfort in your knee as it rests on the floor, move to The Lunge Stretch II.

point of interest The Lunge Stretch is a static stretch; it is not traditional but it is invaluable as a tool for beginners after The Leg Circles.

THE LUNGE STRETCH I

Kneel on all fours, like a cat. Lift your right knee up and forward, placing your right foot forward on the floor in front of you. Keeping your hands on either side of your feet, squeeze your left buttock and push your hips forward into a lunge. Your right shinbone needs to be at a 90-degree angle to the floor, so that your kneecap lines up with your ankle joint. This attention to detail in alignment prevents any undue stress on your right knee.

Draw your navel towards your spine and breathe in and out slowly and naturally six times as you hold the stretch.

Repetitions: One. (Continue on to The Lunge Stretch II before repeating the entire sequence with your left foot forward.)

THE LUNGE STRETCH II

Continuing on from The Lunge Stretch I, place the ball of your left foot on the floor and lift your back knee off the floor. Holding your navel firmly towards your spine to support your back, press your shoulders down towards your hips, stabilising your shoulder girdle and visualising a long, straight line from the crown of your head to your left heel. ②

Breathe in and out slowly and naturally six times as you hold the stretch.

Repetitions: One. (Repeat the entire sequence with your left foot forward.)

*To find our
true balance
we must
honour our
body's position
in equal
proportion.*

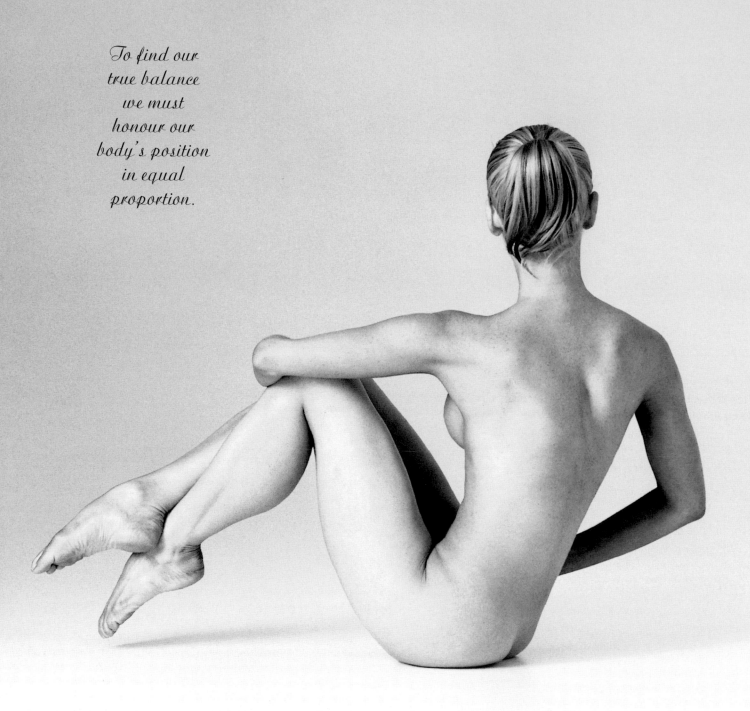

rolling like a ball

focus Balance, control and spinal massage.

imagery Visualise rolling your body into a ball.

precaution Ensure your mat is well padded for comfort. Stop the exericse if you experience any lower-back discomfort.

tip As you roll back and forward your spine should roll smoothly and evenly. Avoid any jarring movements that happen if you have a stiff back or you straighten your spine as you roll.

THE C-CURVE

focus Establishing the C-curve in preparation for Rolling Like a Ball.

Sit tall, with your legs in front of you. Stretch your spine up out of your pelvis, align your shoulders over your hips, bend your legs at a 90-degree angle at the knee joint and hold onto the back of your thighs. Draw your navel to your spine, tighten your abdominals and lift your pelvic floor muscles up towards your ribs.

Breathe in to prepare.

As you breathe out, lower your chin, soften your chest and curve your navel behind your hips, tucking in your pelvis and creating a lengthened letter C from the tip of your head to the base of your spine. ①

Breathe into the back of your lungs and side of your ribs as you hold the C-curve position.

As you breathe out, slowly lengthen up, vertebra by vertebra, starting from the base of your spine and elongating up towards the crown of your head until your back is straight. Finish with your shoulders down and your chest open.

Repetitions: Three. »

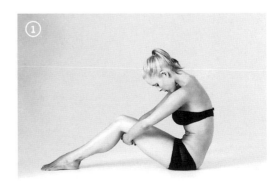

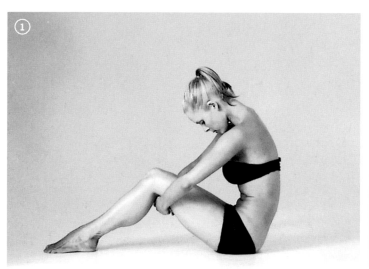

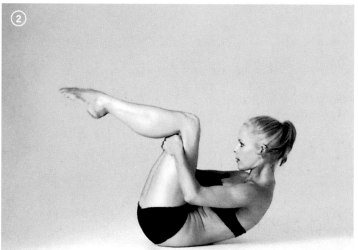

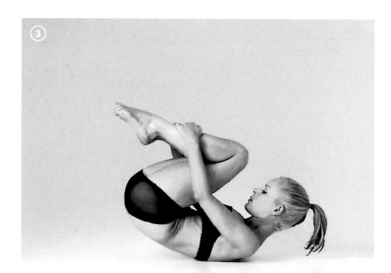

ROLLING LIKE A BALL

Sit in the C-curve position, with your eye-line on your pelvis. ①

Lift your feet and legs off the floor and lean back to a point of balance behind your tailbone. Wrap one hand under each thigh and hold the position.

Breathe in as you roll back onto your shoulder blades, maintaining a C-curve and keeping your shoulders, neck and head off the floor. ②

Keeping your feet off the floor, breathe out and roll back up to the start position.

Repetitions: Ten.

Sit in the C-curve position, with your eye-line on your pelvis. ①

Lift your feet and legs off the floor and lean back to a point of balance behind your tailbone. Wrap one hand over the front of each ankle.

Breathe in as you roll back onto your shoulder blades, maintaining a C-curve and keeping your shoulders, neck and head off the floor. ③

Keeping your feet off the floor, breathe out as you roll up to the start position. (The more tightly you keep your heels towards your hips, the more intensely your abdominals will work to bring you up.)

Repetitions: Ten.

the single-leg stretch

focus Abdominals.

imagery Think of your extended toes reaching towards the furthest point ahead, creating an open pocket of space at the front of your hip.

precaution If you experience discomfort in the back of your neck, support your head with your hands or place your head on the floor. Stop if your lower back feels uncomfortable or weak.

Lie on your back, with your chest curled forward and your legs in a tabletop position (90 degrees at the hip and knee). Point your feet, place your hands gently on top of your knees, anchor your tailbone and draw your navel firmly towards your spine. ①

Breathe in to prepare.

As you breathe out, extend your left leg out straight, keeping the toes of both feet on the same plane and your hands gently holding onto your right knee. ②

As you breathe in, draw your left leg back into the tabletop position.

Repetitions: Five alternating to each side.

variation **a** **s**

As you breathe in, extend your left leg out, then take it back.

As you breathe out, extend your right leg out, then take it back.

Repetitions: Ten alternating to each side.

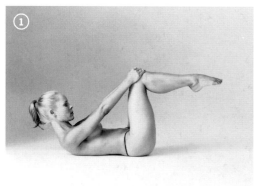

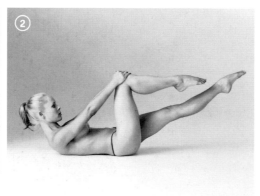

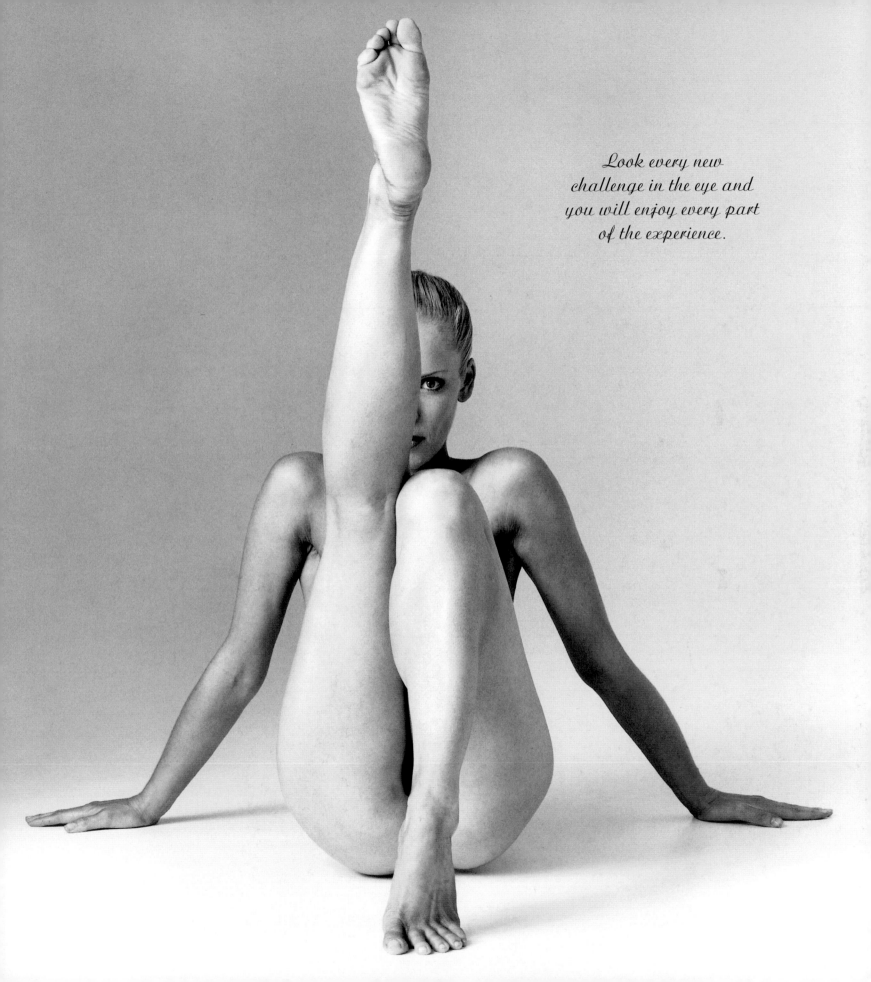

Look every new challenge in the eye and you will enjoy every part of the experience.

the double-leg stretch

focus Abdominals.

imagery Having that great, big stretch in bed when you wake up in the morning.

precaution If you experience discomfort in the back of your neck, support your head with your hands or place your head on the floor. Stop if your lower back feels uncomfortable or weak.

b **i** **a** **s**

Lie on your back, with your chest curled forward and your legs in a tabletop position (90 degrees at the hip and knee). Point your feet, place your hands gently on top of your knees, anchor your tailbone and draw your navel firmly towards your spine. ①

As you breathe in, simultaneously stretch your arms back by your ears and extend both legs out straight, at an angle at which you can safely keep your back imprinted into the floor. (The lower your legs, the more advanced the exercise.) ②

As you breathe out, gracefully circle your arms around your sides and bring your knees back to the tabletop position, once again resting your hands on your knees. ③

Repetitions: Ten.

variation **a** **s**

Continuing on, reverse the circle of your arms by reaching them out to your sides and back by your ears as you breathe in. Bring your arms over your head and back towards your knees as you breathe out.

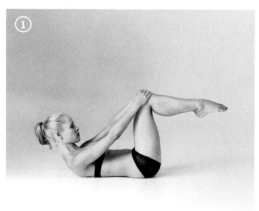

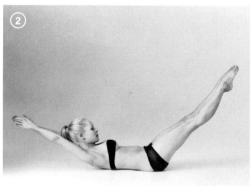

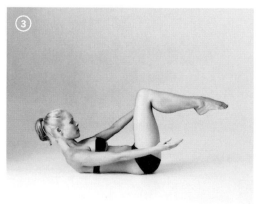

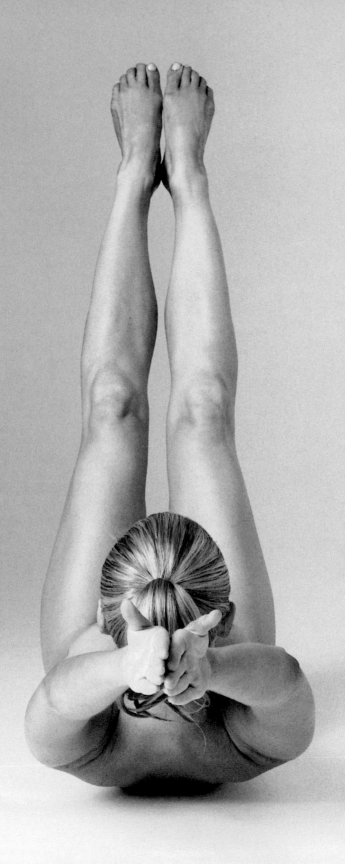

As you reach your arms behind you and your legs forward, contemplate how what is behind us is the foundation on which we build our future.

the hamstring pull

focus Abdominals and pelvic stability.

imagery Visualise your legs crisscrossing like a pair of scissors.

precaution If you experience discomfort in the back of your neck, support your head with your hands or place your head on the floor. Stop if your lower back feels uncomfortable or weak.

tip The more slowly you do this exercise, the more control you will have over your pelvis.

Lie on your back, with your chest curled forward and your legs stretched straight up towards the ceiling. Point your feet and place your hands gently behind your thighs, keeping your tailbone anchored. Draw your navel firmly towards your spine, narrowing your waist.

Breathe in to prepare.

As you breathe out, place both hands on the back of your right thigh and, keeping your right leg vertical, tighten the back of your left thigh and extend it down until it is a little way from the floor. Keep your pelvis strong and stable in its neutral position.

As you breathe in, draw your left leg back to its start position.

Repetitions: Five alternating to each side.

variation

To challenge your pelvic stability, add a small pulse and extra breath out (known as percussive breathing) to both legs.

variation

Ten repetitions alternating to each side.

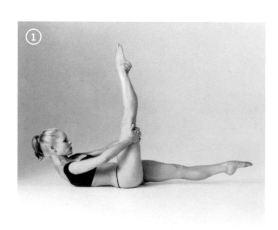

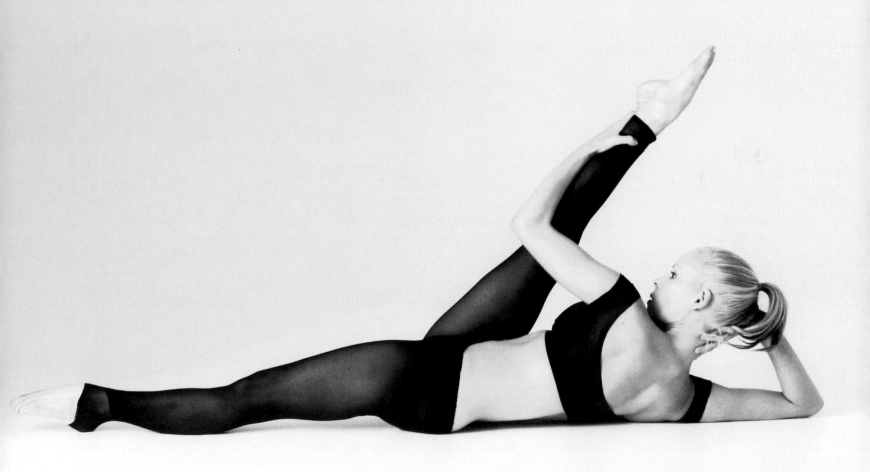

Mastering and disciplining our most intrinsic movements allows us the freedom to explore our body's greater depths.

the double-leg lowers

focus Abdominals and hip dissociation.

imagery Visualise your legs as a door swinging on its hinges and your torso as the strong and stable doorframe.

precaution Stop if your lower back feels uncomfortable or weak.

PREPARATION: THE DOUBLE-LEG EXTENSION

Lie on your back, with your chest curled forward and your legs in a tabletop position (90 degrees at the hip and knee). Point your feet, anchor your tailbone and draw your navel firmly towards your spine. Keeping your elbows open, place your hands behind your head and link your fingers together, with your thumbs working down the back of your neck. ①

Breathe in to prepare.

As you breathe out, extend both legs out straight, at an angle at which you can safely keep your back imprinted into the floor. (The lower your legs, the more advanced the exercise.) ②

As you breathe in, bring your legs back into the tabletop position, keeping your tailbone anchored.

Repetitions: Ten.

DOUBLE-LEG LOWERS

Lie on your back, with your chest curled forward, your legs straight up (90 degrees at the hip) and your feet pointed. Keeping your elbows open, place your hands behind your head and link your fingers together, with your thumbs working down the back of your neck. ②

Anchor your tailbone and turn your legs out, placing your heels together and your toes apart in a V position. Draw your navel firmly towards your spine, narrowing your waist.

Breathe in to prepare.

As you breathe out, squeeze your buttocks and lower your legs as close to the floor as possible without moving your lower back or pelvis. (The lower your legs, the more advanced the exercise.)

As you breathe in, anchor your tailbone and lift your legs back up to the start position.

Repetitions: Ten.

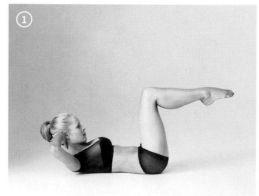

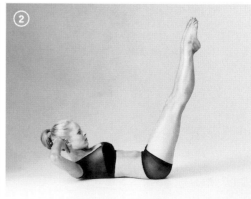

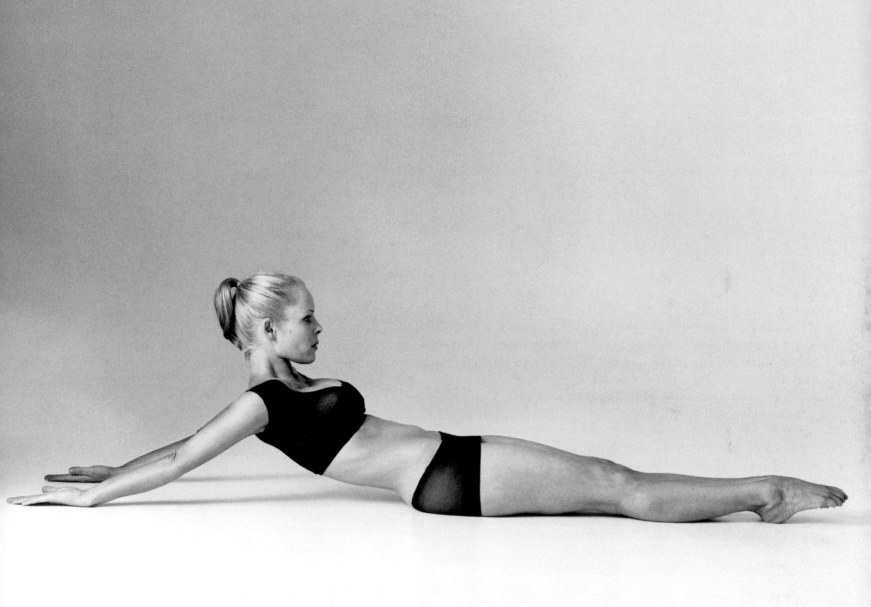

To truly experience the moment, we must be truly present in it.

the single-leg stretch twist

focus The sides of your abdominals.

precaution Stop if your lower back feels uncomfortable or weak.

Lie on your back, with your chest curled forward and your legs in a tabletop position (90 degrees at the hip and knee). Point your feet, anchor your tailbone and draw your navel firmly towards your spine. Keeping your elbows open, place your hands behind your head and link your fingers together, with your thumbs working down the back of your neck. ①

Breathe in to prepare.

Holding your hips still and stable and your elbows open, breathe out as you draw the back of your left shoulder forward towards your right knee and simultaneously extend your left leg out straight, with the toes of both feet remaining on the same plane. ②

As you breathe in, draw your left leg back into the tabletop position and bring your chest through centre, keeping the curl in your upper back.

Repetitions: Five alternating to each side.

Lie on your back, with your chest curled forward and your legs in a tabletop position (90 degrees at the hip and knee). Point your feet, anchor your tailbone and draw your navel firmly towards your spine. Keeping your elbows open, place your hands behind your head and link your fingers together, with your thumbs working down the back of your neck. ①

As you breathe in, draw the back of your left shoulder forward towards your right knee and simultaneously extend your left leg out straight, with the toes of both feet remaining on the same plane. ② Return to centre.

As you breathe out, draw the back of your right shoulder forward towards your left knee and simultaneously extend your right leg out straight, with the toes of both feet remaining on the same plane, then return to centre.

Repetitions: Ten alternating to each side.

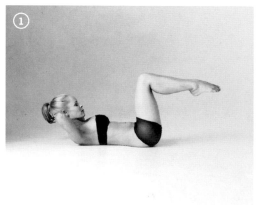 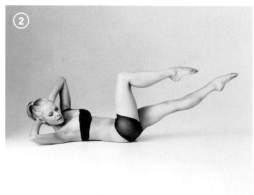

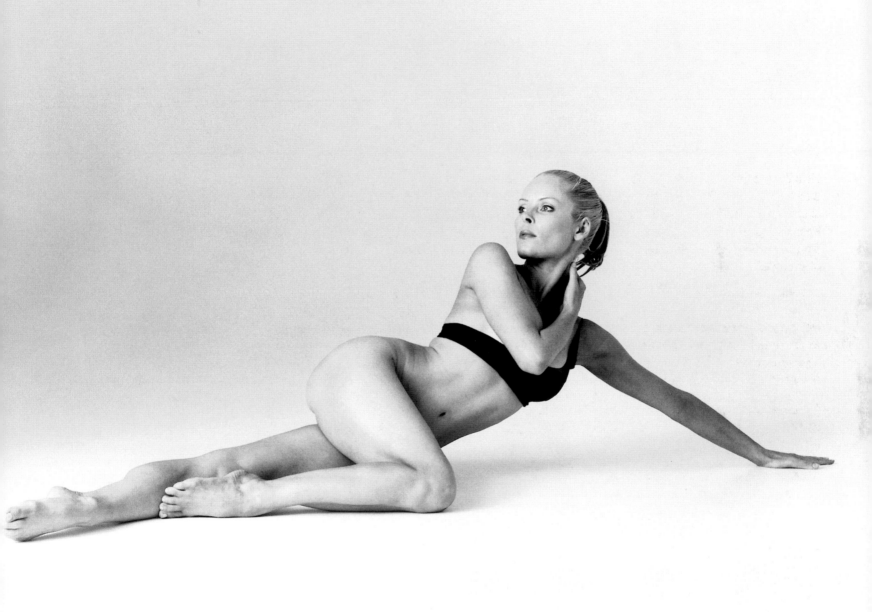

When we centre our thoughts we are able to move forward with integrity.

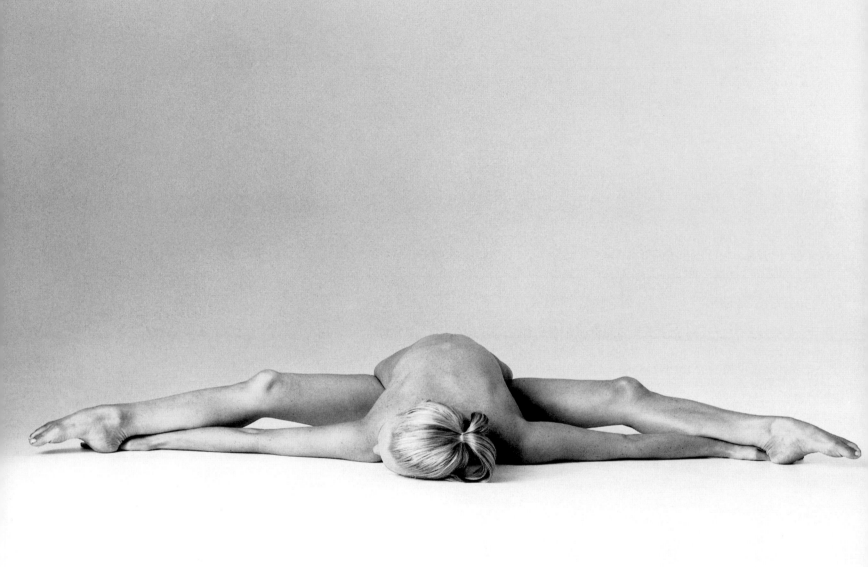

The responsibility for developing our mind and body begins and ends with our self.

the spine stretch

focus Spinal flexion and mobilisation using spine extensors and the seated posture (a co-contraction of the abdominals and spine extensors).

imagery Visualise yourself in the surf, diving under a big wave heading out to sea – you curl your upper body over and reach your fingertips down and forward into the water, then as you come up you extend your spine to resurface.

Sit up straight, with your pelvis in neutral (hip bones and pubic bone on the same vertical plane) and your legs stretched straight out, a little wider than your shoulders, with your feet flexed. Stretch your arms out in front (between your legs), with your fingertips touching the floor.

Breathe in to prepare.

As you breathe out, drop your chin softly towards your chest and roll each vertebra forward one by one, keeping your lower back straight and your pelvis in neutral, and sliding your fingertips along the floor. ①

Hold the upper-back stretch, with your navel drawn firmly towards your spine, and breathe in through the back of your lungs and the sides of your ribs.

As you breathe out, roll your spine, vertebra by vertebra, back into the start position.

Repetitions: Three.

Continuing on, place your hands comfortably on your thighs.

Breathe in to prepare.

As you breathe out, drop your chin softly towards your chest and roll each vertebra forward one by one, keeping your lower back straight and your pelvis in neutral, and sliding your hands down your legs towards your ankles.

Breathe in through the back of your lungs and the sides of your ribs, and as you hold onto your legs, draw your spine forward into a straight, long diagonal line, with your shoulders pulled back into place and your chest open. ②

》

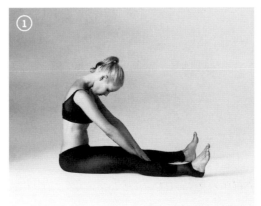

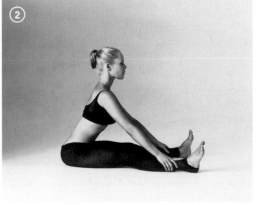

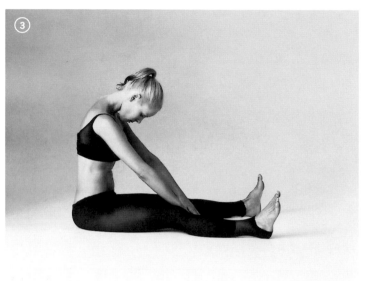

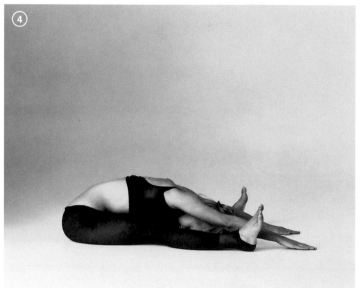

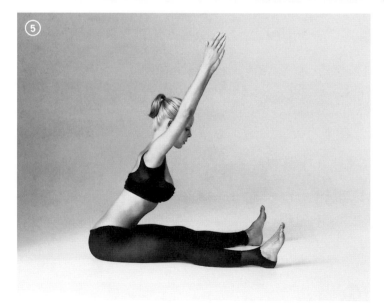

As you breathe out, draw your navel back towards your spine and, curving your upper back once more, return your pelvis to its neutral position.

As you breathe in, continue to roll your spine back up, vertebra by vertebra, until you are sitting straight, allowing your hands to slide back into the start position.

Repetitions: Three.

  s

Sit up straight, with your pelvis in neutral (hip bones and pubic bone on the same vertical plane), your legs stretched straight out, a little wider than your shoulders, with your feet flexed. Stretch your arms out in front at chest height, parallel to the floor with palms face-down.

Breathe in to prepare.

As you breathe out, drop your chin softly towards your chest and curl your upper back over, vertebra by vertebra, keeping your lower back straight and your pelvis in neutral. Keeping your shoulders relaxed, reach your fingertips down towards the floor. ③

As you breathe in, stretch your fingers forward along the floor, lowering your spine as close to the floor as you can, stretching out the back of your legs and your spine. ④

Drawing your torso forward, lift it into a straight, long, diagonal line, with your arms up by your ears, palms facing towards each other. ⑤

As you breathe out, curve your spine over again, reach forward with your arms, sliding your fingertips along the floor, and draw your pelvis back into its neutral position.

As you breathe in, unravel your spine, vertebra by vertebra, to return to the start position.

Repetitions: Four.

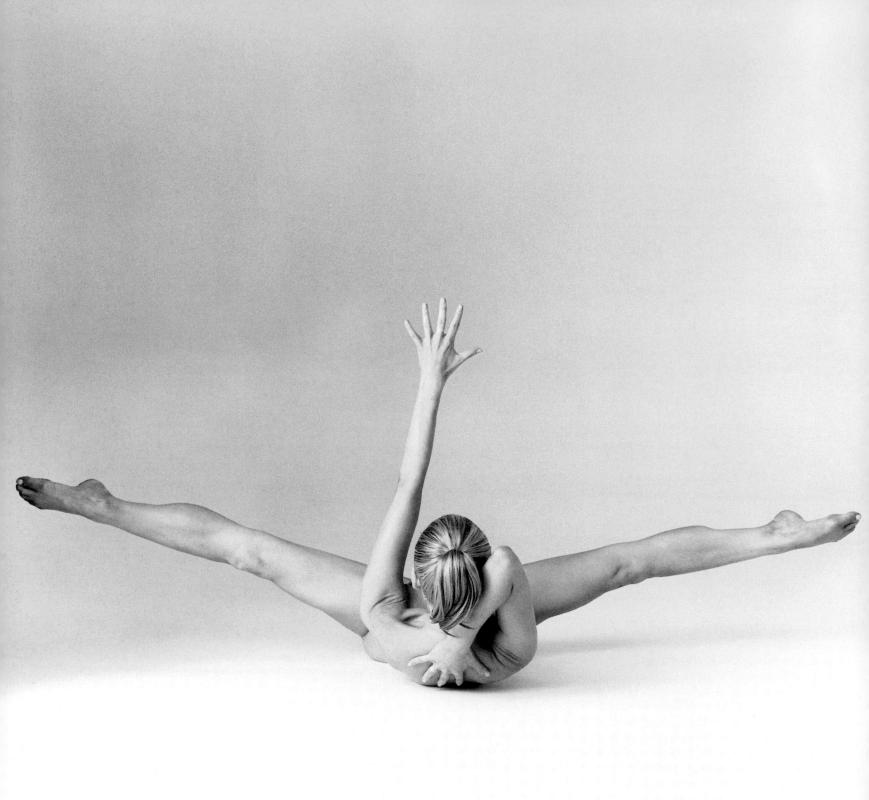

Visualise what you want to achieve and have the patience to follow through with your vision.

the open-leg rocker

focus Balance, control, spinal massage, and abdominal and spinal-extensor strength, to maintain a long, stable back in the straight position.

imagery Visualise yourself sitting in a rocking chair, smoothly rolling forward and backwards.

modification If you are unable to maintain a straight back when you lengthen your legs, reach your arms around your legs and hold on underneath your thighs.

THE OPEN-LEG BALANCE

Sit up straight, with your legs in a diamond position (knees bent up and open, big toes touching), your arms on the inside of your legs and your hands holding onto your ankles. Maintaining a straight spine with your shoulders open and down, lean back and lift your feet just off the floor. ①

As you breathe in, extend your left leg out a little wider than your shoulder, keeping your shoulders down, your pelvis square and your spine long and straight. ②

As you breathe out, return to the start position.

Repetitions: Two with each leg.

As you breathe in, extend both legs a little wider than your shoulders, keeping your shoulders down, your spine long and straight, your pelvis square and your chest open. ③

As you breathe out, return to the start position.

Repetitions: Four.

»

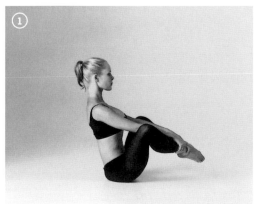

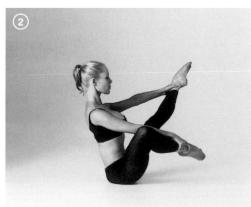

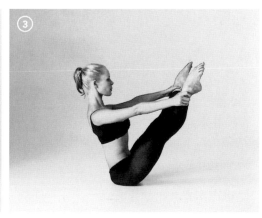

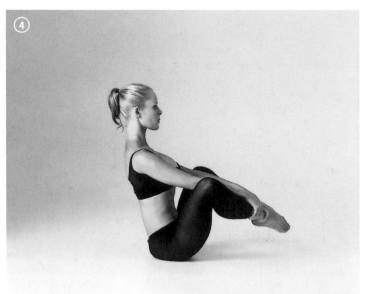

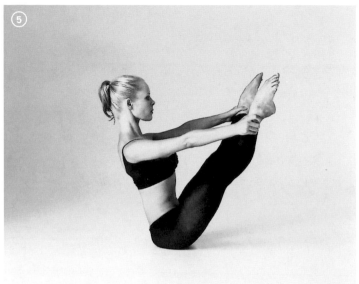

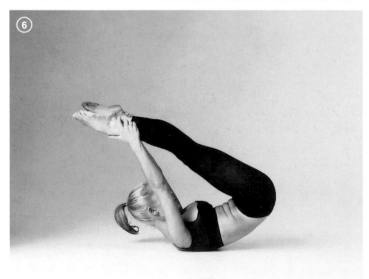

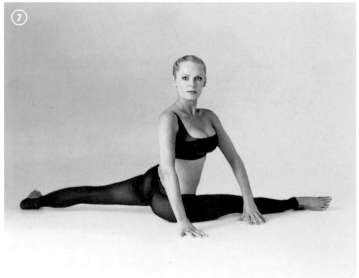

Continuing on from the beginner variation, hold your start position. ④

Breathe in as you extend both legs a little wider than your shoulders, keeping your spine long and straight, your shoulders down, your pelvis square and your chest open. ⑤

As you breathe out, return to the start position. ④

Keeping your eye-line on your pelvis, breathe in as you roll back onto your shoulder blades in a C-curve, keeping your shoulders, neck and head off the floor.

As you breathe out, roll back up to the start position.

Repetitions: Four.

a

Continuing on from the intermediate variation, breathe in as you extend both legs a little wider than your shoulders. ⑤

Breathe out as you hold your position.

Keeping your eye-line on your pelvis and your legs straight, breathe in as you roll back onto your shoulder blades in a C-curve, keeping your shoulders, neck and head off the floor. ⑥

As you breathe out, roll back up to the start position with your legs straight.

Repetitions: Ten.

Breathing at a relaxed pace, with your navel drawn towards your spine, hold the start position and let go of your legs while maintaining the pose with control. Slowly lower your legs to the floor in a comfortable V position, ready for The Split Stretch.

THE SPLIT STRETCH

focus Lengthening the hip flexors after The Open-leg Rocker, and rotation of the spine to increase the suppleness of the torso.

Imagery As you are sitting tall, visualise the crown of your head reaching towards the ceiling.

precaution If you feel any discomfort in your lower back during the rotation, ease into a more comfortable position.

tip You need to sit very tall for this exercise, with your pelvis in neutral and your legs forward in a V position. If you have difficulty getting your pelvis into a neutral position because your lower back, buttocks or legs are tight, sit on a rolled-up towel that is high enough for you to achieve the ideal position.

Sit tall, with your legs forward in a V position and your pelvis in neutral (hip bones and pubic bone on the same vertical plane). Flex your feet and keep your arms relaxed by your sides.

Breathing naturally, rotate your body to the right, rolling your left thigh in and using the inside part of your left flexed foot to push into the floor to facilitate your hip-flexor stretch. Place your hands wherever they feel comfortable to support you, and look behind you to increase the rotational stretch of your spine. ⑦

Repetitions: Two alternating to each side.

the pendulum

focus Rotation and abdominals.

imagery Visualise your chest as a lead weight, enabling you to keep your chest still while moving your lower body freely to facilitate an effective chest and ribcage stretch.

precaution If you feel any discomfort in your lower back, bend your legs into the tabletop position (90 degrees at hip and knee) and revert to The Side to Side exercise (see page 44).

Lie on your back, with your arms stretched out to the sides of your body at chest height and your palms face-down. Point your feet and lift your legs straight up, with a 90-degree angle at your hips. Squeeze your inner thighs together and keep your toes on the same plane. Draw your navel firmly towards your spine and anchor your tailbone. Use your abdominals and the back of your ribs to keep your spine flat to the floor.

Breathe in to prepare.

Anchoring your left shoulder and shoulder blade, breathe out as you roll your head to the left and carry both legs over to the right, allowing your hips, waist and ribs to follow gracefully. Indulge in the stretch behind your ribcage and at the front of your chest. ①

As you breathe in, use your abdominals to draw your ribs, waist, hips and legs back to the start position, rolling your head back to centre.

Repetitions: Three alternating to each side.

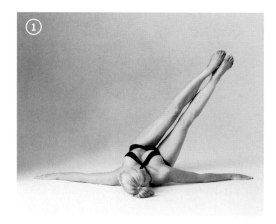

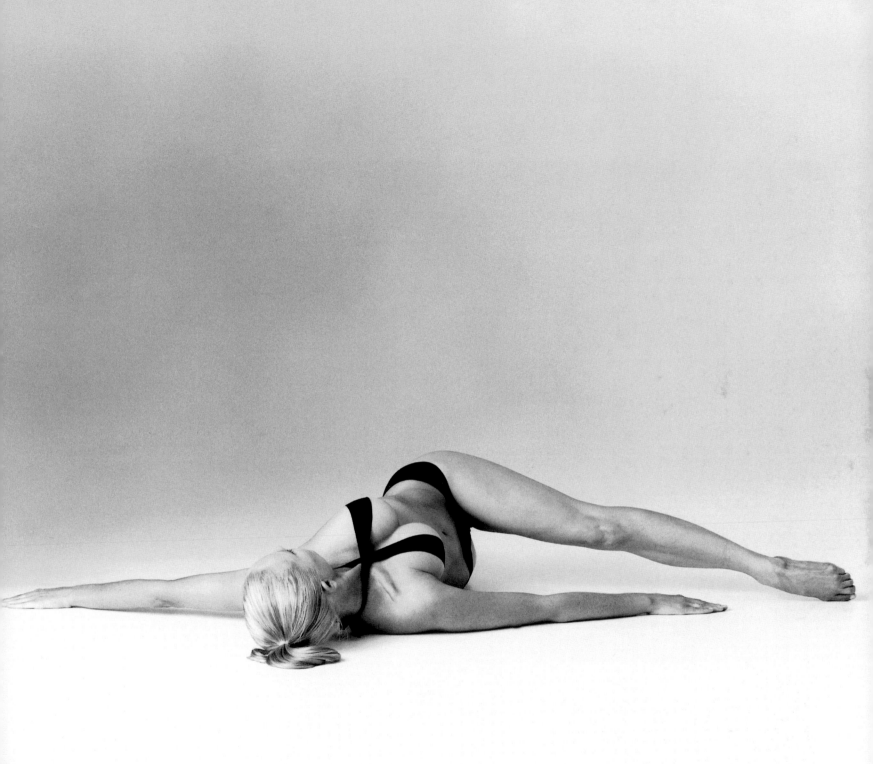

Our body, like life, is in a constant state of change, and we must respect its journey.

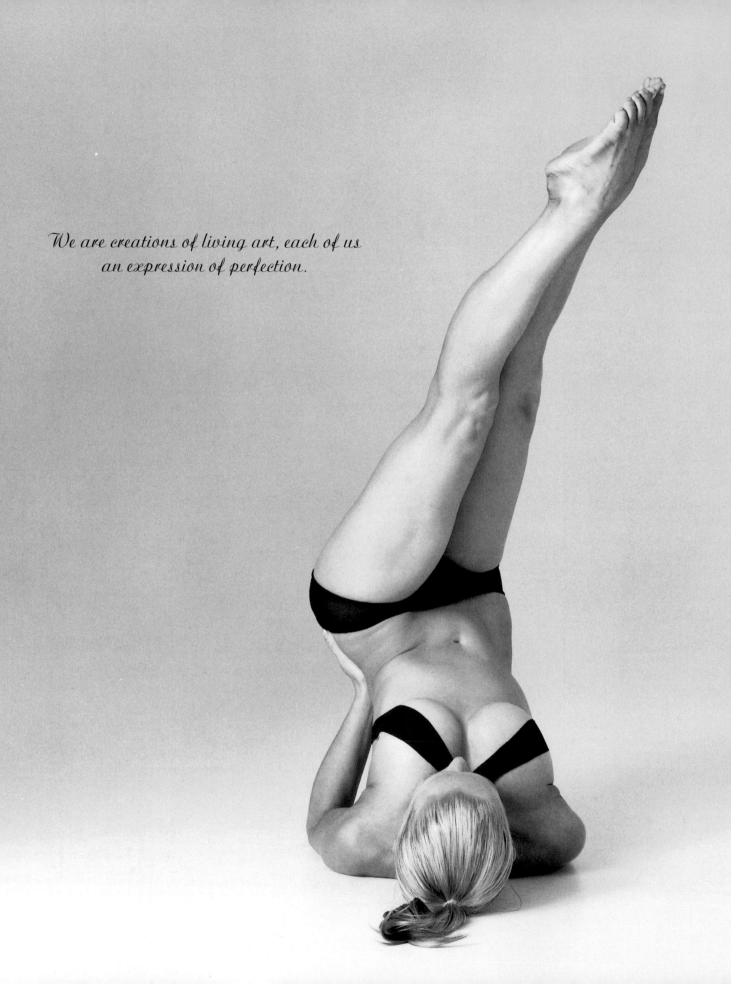

We are creations of living art, each of us an expression of perfection.

the corkscrew

focus Balance, core control and spinal articulation.

imagery Visualise your legs moving in the action of a cowboy's lasso.

precaution Stop if you have any lower-back discomfort. The advanced version should be performed for the first time under experienced supervision.

tip Begin with small leg circles, focusing on your form. As you grow stronger, make your circles bigger.

Lie on your back, with your arms stretched out to the sides of your body at chest height, with your palms face-down. Point your feet and lift your legs straight up. Anchor your tailbone and narrow your waist. Draw your navel firmly towards your spine, and use your abdominals and the back of your ribs to keep your spine flat on the floor.

Breathe in to prepare.

Squeezing your inner thighs together, anchor your left shoulder and shoulder blade. As you breathe out, lower your legs over to the right, keeping your toes on the same plane and allowing your left hip to lift. ①

Following a circle, continue moving your legs towards the floor, and maintain a stable spine as you return your pelvis to neutral and bring your hip squarely back to the floor.

As you breathe in, complete the circle, keeping your right shoulder and shoulder blade anchored to the floor. ②

Repetitions: Three alternating each way.

»

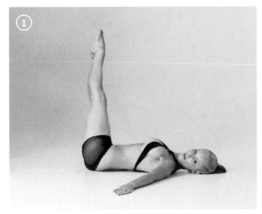

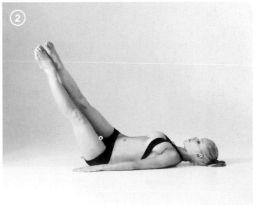

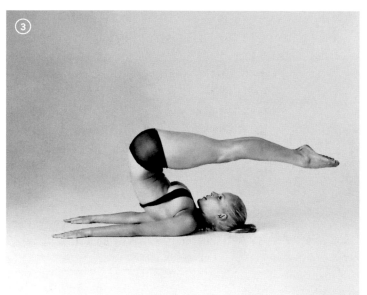

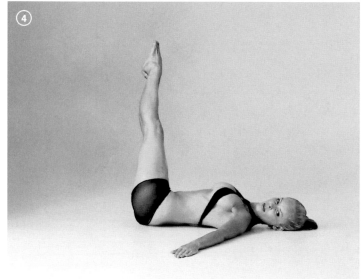

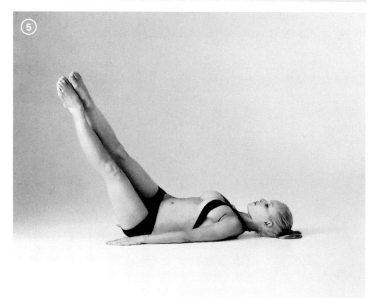

prerequisite Only attempt the advanced version if you are strong and competent at The Roll-over (see page 63) and the intermediate variation of The Corkscrew (see page 95).

Lie on your back, with your arms stretched out to the sides of your body at chest height, with your palms face-down. Point your feet and lift your legs straight up. Anchor your tailbone and narrow your waist. Draw your navel firmly towards your spine, and use your abdominals and the back of your ribs to keep your spine flat on the floor.

Breathe in to prepare.

As you breathe out, focus on using your abdominals to carry your legs over your head until they finish parallel to the floor and your body weight is balanced between your shoulder blades. ③

As you breathe in, lift your left hip towards your left rib, carrying both legs over to the right.

As you breathe out, roll down the right side of your back, following a circle as you lower your legs down. ④ Continue to circle your legs, allowing your pelvis to roll through neutral as your legs lower towards the floor.

As you breathe in, continue to move your legs over to the left. ⑤ Roll up the left side of your back, finishing in The Roll-over position, with your legs behind you parallel to the floor, and your right hip lifted towards your right ribs.

As you breathe out, centre your hips, balancing your body weight on the back of your shoulder blades. ③

Repetitions: Three alternating each way.

the saw

focus Spinal rotation, stretching the back of the shoulder and ribs, and abdominal and spinal-extensor strength to maintain a long, stable back in the straight position.

imagery Visualise your sit bones and pelvis glued to the floor, allowing freedom of movement in your upper body to facilitate the ideal stretch.

tip You need to sit very tall for this exercise, with your pelvis in neutral and your legs forward in a V position. If you have difficulty getting your pelvis into a neutral position because your lower back, buttocks or legs are tight, sit on a rolled-up towel that is high enough for you to achieve the ideal position.

Sit tall, with your pelvis in neutral (hip bones and pubic bone on the same vertical plane) and your legs stretched out in front of you; visualise a straight line running down the centre of your body. Move both legs out 45 degrees from centre and flex your feet. Stretch your arms out to the sides of your body, parallel to the floor at chest height, palms face-down. Visualise the crown of your head reaching towards the ceiling and your torso and arms sandwiched between two panes of glass. ①

Keeping your hips and sit bones anchored, breathe in as you twist your body towards your right, keeping your torso and arms aligned and visualising the panes of glass.

As you breathe out, reach your chest forward over your right thigh, sliding the back of your left palm down the outside of your right leg and reaching out towards (and even past) your smallest toe. Use the pressure of palm against leg to assist in increasing your twist and stretch, holding your torso as close to the floor as possible. Reach your right arm behind you, allowing your thumb to rotate naturally towards the floor and your head and eye-line to look back, with your left ear listening to your right thigh. ②

As you breathe in, straighten your back to an upright position, maintaining your spinal rotation.

As you breathe out, return to the start position.

Repetitions: Five alternating to each side.

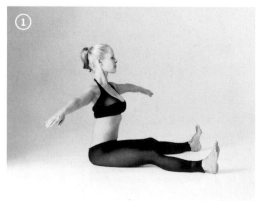

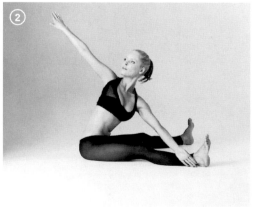

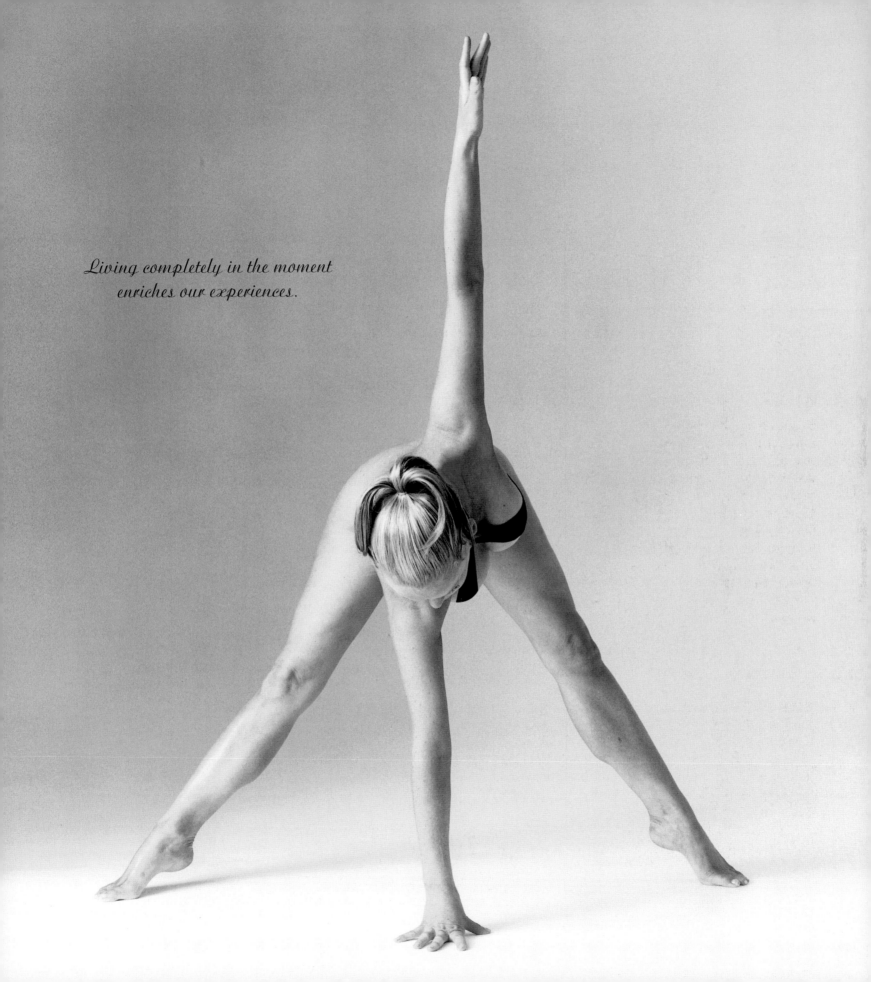

Living completely in the moment enriches our experiences.

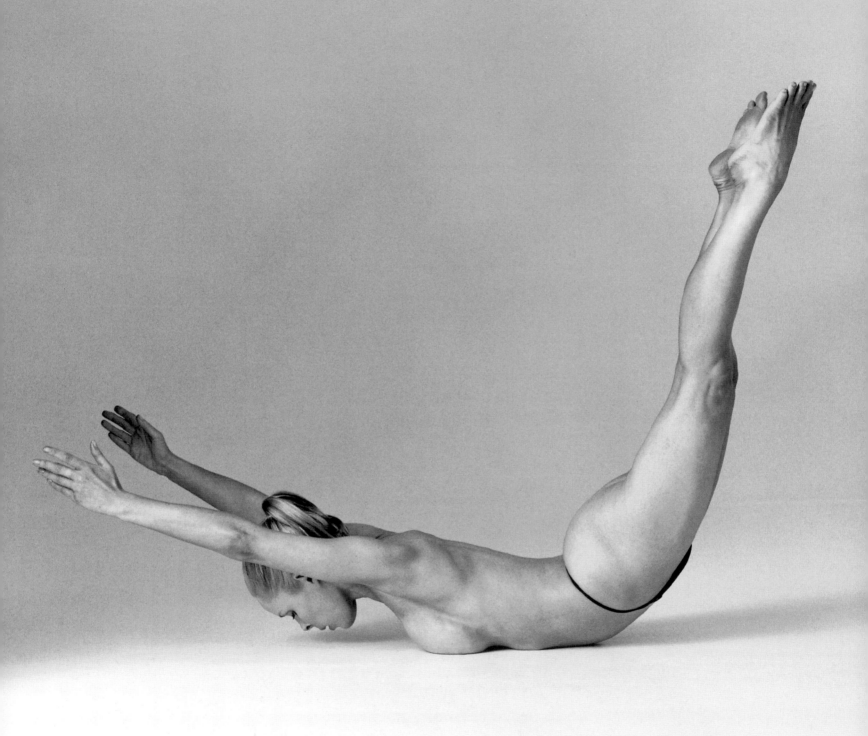

As you extend your body to greater challenge, open your heart with abandon, trusting in the wisdom of your intuition.

the swan dive

focus Spinal extension and abdominal stretch.

imagery Visualise your body moving fluidly like a rocking horse.

precaution If you feel any lower-back discomfort, stop the exercise and sit back on your heels in The Rest Position (see page 108).

tip To begin, keep your elbows on the floor, limiting your range of movement. As you become more adept at this exercise, lift your elbows and spine further, careful to only extend as far as is comfortable. Be aware that the maximum flexibility of the spine in extension is individual, so work safely within your own physical ability.

Lie face-down. Place your arms in a goal-post position, with your elbows resting on the floor slightly beneath shoulder height and your hands approximately head height, your forearms parallel to your body. Align your pelvis in the neutral position (hip bones and pubic bone on the same plane). Draw your navel towards your spine, narrowing your waist, and lift your pelvic floor muscles to support your lower back. Gently squeeze your lower buttocks to assist in keeping your pubic bone anchored.

Breathe in to prepare.

As you breathe out, push into your palms and elbows, lifting your upper back off the floor and extending your spine, taking care to extend only as far as is comfortable. Visualise the crown of your head reaching

forward as it lifts, lengthening the space between each vertebra of your spine, your neck in line with the graceful curve of your back. ①

As you breathe in, lower your upper body to the floor, maintaining a strong abdominal wall and lengthening through each vertebra of your spine.

Keeping your pelvis in neutral, your lower buttocks firm and your arms in goal-post position, breathe out as you lift both legs slightly off the floor, lengthening through the front of your thighs and reaching your toes as far away from your hips as possible. ②

As you breathe in, return your legs to the start position.

Repetitions: Five. »

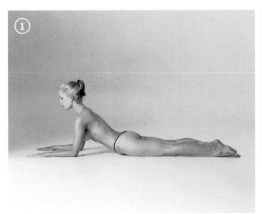

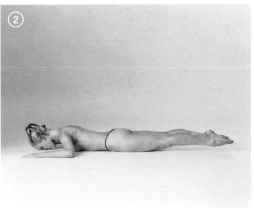

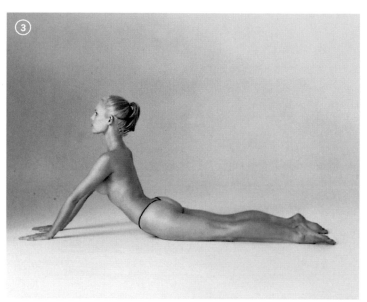

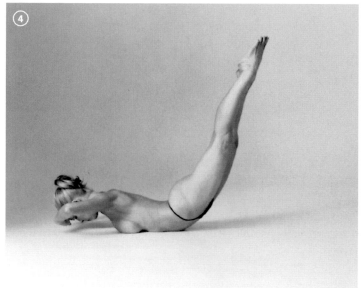

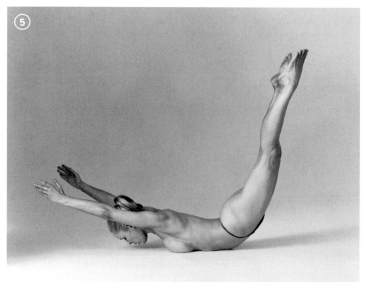

This exercise is inappropriate for anyone with a lower-back issue and should be performed for the first time under experienced supervision.

Lie face-down. Place your arms in a goal-post position, with your elbows resting on the floor slightly beneath shoulder height and your hands approximately head height, your forearms parallel to your body. Align your pelvis in the neutral position (hip bones and pubic bone on the same plane). Draw your navel towards your spine, narrowing your waist, and lift your pelvic floor muscles to support your lower back. Gently squeeze your lower buttocks to assist in keeping your pubic bone anchored.

Breathe in to prepare.

As you breathe out, push into your palms and lift your upper back and elbows off the floor, taking care to extend only as far as is comfortable. Visualise the crown of your head reaching forward as it lifts, lengthening the space between each vertebra of your spine, your neck in line with the graceful curve of your back. ③

As you breathe in, simultaneously swing your legs up (visualising your toes reaching up to the ceiling) and bring your arms forward in a diamond-shaped position, gently connecting the back of your palms with your forehead. ④

As you breathe out, smoothly return your upper body to the start position and return your legs to the floor.

Repetitions: Five to ten sets.

This exercise is inappropriate for anyone with a lower-back issue and should be performed for the first time under experienced supervision.

Lie face-down. Place your arms in a goal-post position, with your elbows resting on the floor slightly beneath shoulder height and your hands approximately head height, your forearms parallel to your body. Align your pelvis in the neutral position (hip bones and pubic bone on the same plane). Draw your navel towards your spine, narrowing your waist, and lift your pelvic floor muscles to support your lower back. Gently squeeze your lower buttocks to assist in keeping your pubic bone anchored.

Breathe in to prepare.

As you breathe out, push into your palms and lift your upper back and elbows off the floor, taking care to extend only as far as is comfortable. Visualise the crown of your head reaching forward as it lifts, lengthening the space between each vertebra of your spine, your neck in line with the graceful curve of your back. ③

As you breathe in, simultaneously swing your legs up (visualising your toes reaching up to the ceiling) with your arms stretched forward and out above your head. ⑤

As you breathe out, keep your arms above your head and swing your body up until your spine is as upright as possible. Visualise your body moving fluidly like a rocking horse between these two movements.

Repetitions: Five to ten sets.

the single-leg kick

focus Spinal extension, pelvic stability and coordination.

imagery Visualise a sling suspended from above, keeping your waist and ribs lifted and drawn back into your spine.

precaution If you feel any lower-back discomfort, try lowering your upper body until it hovers just off the floor, and move your arms into a diamond position. If this change is unsuccessful, stop the exercise and move into The Rest Position (see page 108) to release your lower back. If you have a knee issue and feel discomfort, stop the exercise.

Lie face-down, with your legs stretched out behind you hip-width apart and your feet pointed. Raise your torso up onto your elbows, with your elbows directly underneath your shoulders, your hands clasped together and your neck continuing the graceful curve of your back. Press your elbows firmly into the floor, allowing you to reach your neck and the crown of your head away from your shoulders. Draw your navel towards your spine and tighten your lower buttocks, stabilising your pelvis.

Breathe in to prepare.

As you breathe out twice in a short, sharp manner (try to engage your abdominals a little harder on each breath out; this is called percussive breathing), kick your left foot back towards your buttocks, adding an extra pulse in the kick to match your percussive breath. ①

As you breathe in, lift and extend your left thigh off the floor, straightening your left leg and using your lower buttocks and abdominals to assist you in maintaining a stable pelvis. ②

Lower your left leg back onto the floor.

Repetitions: Five each side.

Continuing on, use strong abdominals and buttocks to maintain a stable pelvis as you lift both legs a little off the floor. Hold the straightened leg up like this as you repeat the exercise, keeping your hamstring and buttocks active. Double the pace of your kicks and percussive breathing.

Repetitions: Five alternating to each side.

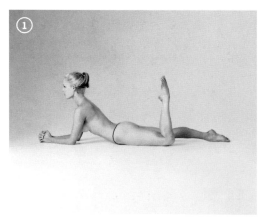 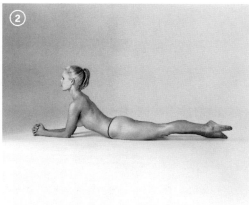

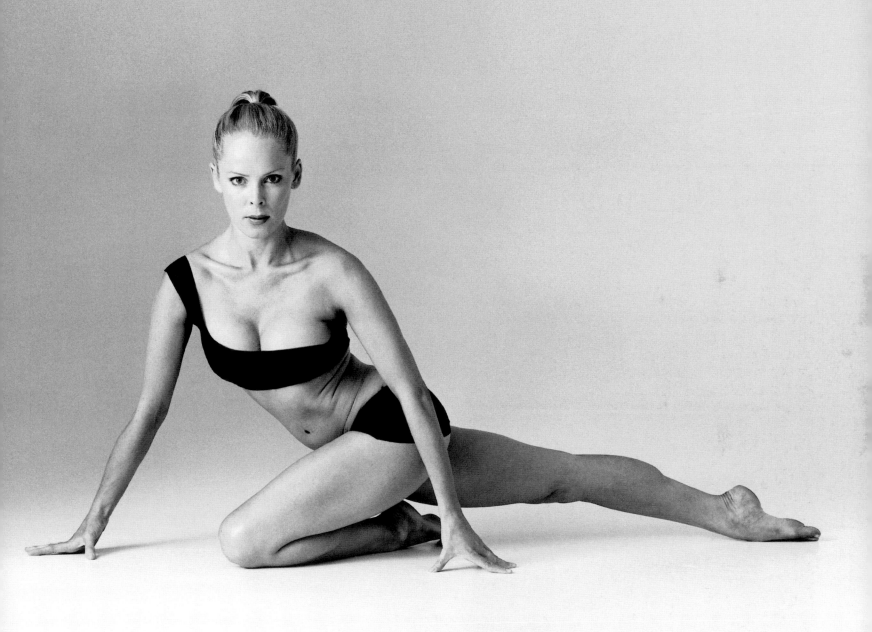

We must each believe in the unlimited potential of our mind, body and spirit.

the double-leg kick

focus Spinal extension and pelvic stability.

imagery As you simultaneously extend your spine and legs, visualise your body as the hull of a sleek boat.

precaution If you feel any lower-back discomfort, stop the exercise and move into The Rest Position (see page 108) to release your spine.

Lie face-down, with your head resting to one side. Clasp your fingers together behind your back and place them on your upper buttocks, applying firm pressure in the direction of your feet. Lengthen your pubic bone down towards the floor until it sits on the same plane as the front of your hipbones (this is your neutral pelvis). Stretch both legs along the floor, hip-width apart, and point your feet. Draw your navel to your spine and tighten your lower gluteals.

Breathe in to prepare.

Hold your pelvis still and stable, and keep your abdominals and lower gluteals firm. Breathe out three times in a short, sharp manner (try to engage your abdominals a little harder on each breath out; this is called percussive breathing) as you kick both feet towards your buttocks with corresponding pulses to match your breathing. ① Use the pressure of your clasped hands on your upper buttocks to assist in maintaining a still pelvis.

As you breathe in, stretch your clasped hands and arms towards your toes, lifting your upper back into extension and straightening your legs a little off the floor, allowing the line of your neck to continue the graceful curve of your back. ②

Repetitions: Ten. (Alternate the side your head rests on for each repetition.)

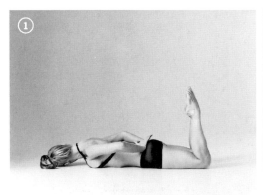

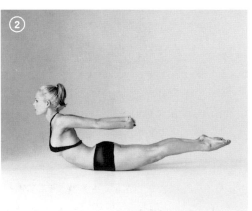

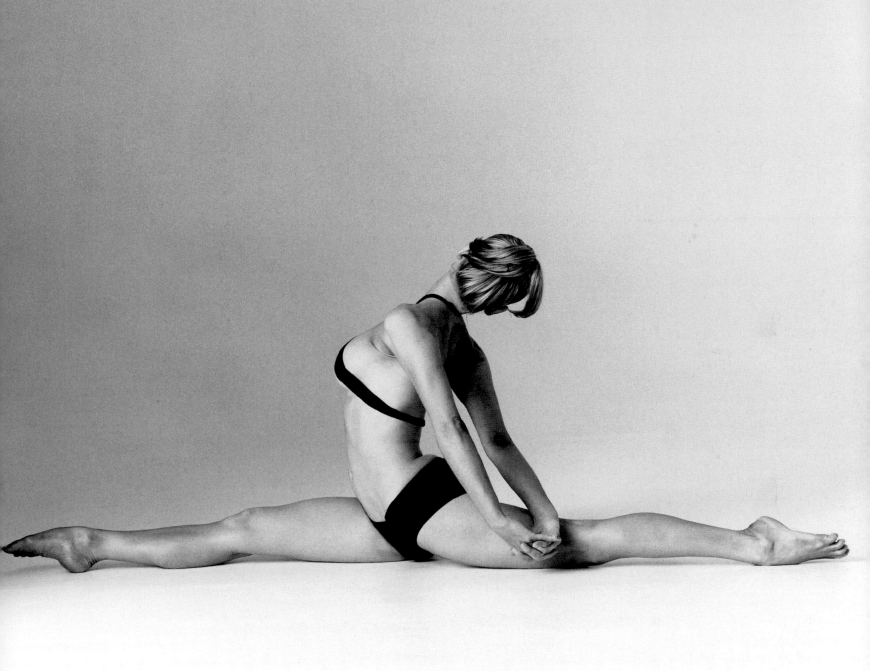

*There is a blissful sense of clarity when we consciously approach each new challenge
with tranquillity and heightened self-awareness.*

the rest position

THE REST POSITION I

focus To release and relax the back.

Sit back on your heels, with your knees slightly apart and your big toes touching. Lean forward until your chest rests on your thighs. Allow both arms to stretch out on the floor in front as your head relaxes gently on the floor. Hold this position for six deep breaths. ①

THE REST POSITION II

focus To release and relax the back.

tip This variation is suitable for people who find the first variation uncomfortable due to a neck or shoulder issue.

Sit back on your heels, with your knees and feet together. Lean forward until your chest rests on your thighs. Allow both arms to lengthen back beside your legs as your head relaxes gently on the floor. Hold this position for six deep breaths. ②

THE REST POSITION III

focus To release and relax the back.

tip This variation is suitable for people who find the first variation uncomfortable due to a knee issue. If you have any difficulty keeping the back of your head or shoulders relaxed on the floor, place a padded towel or small cushion behind your head.

Lie on your back hugging both knees towards your chest, with your fingers interlocked between the back of your calves and thighs. Softly lower your chin towards your throat, lengthening your neck. Hold this position for six deep breaths. ③

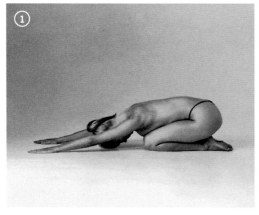
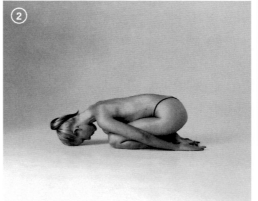
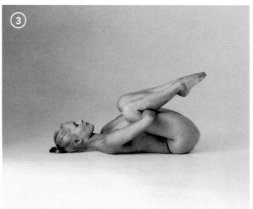

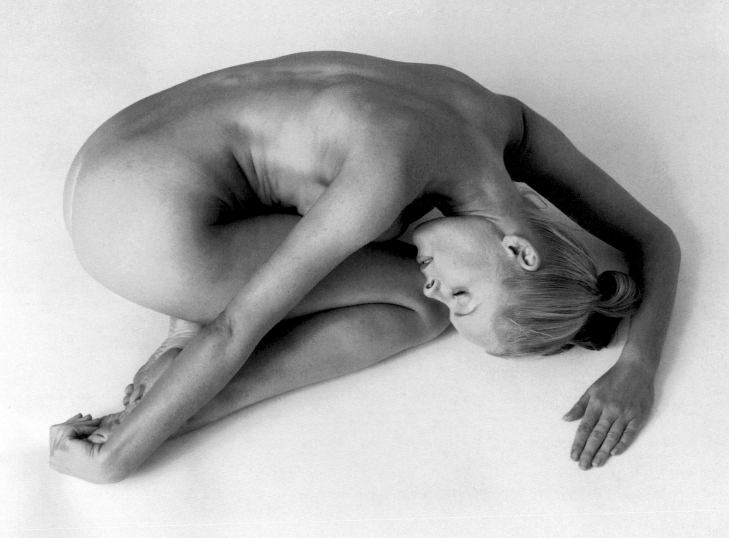

In times of great mental and physical challenge, we must learn to appreciate listening to the silence.

the neck pull

focus Spinal articulation, coordination and integration between the abdominals and hip flexors.

imagery Visualise your lower body cemented into the ground and each vertebra in your spine peeling off the floor one at a time smoothly and gracefully.

prerequisite Only attempt this exercise if you are strong and competent at The Roll-up (see page 59).

precaution Stop if you feel any lower-back discomfort.

Lie on your back, with your legs stretched out flat along the floor hip-width apart, with your feet flexed. Place your hands behind your head and link your fingers together, with your thumbs working down the back of your neck. Draw your navel firmly towards your spine and relax your ribcage and shoulders. Keep your elbows open for the entire exercise (this will make this exercise significantly harder than The Roll-up).

Breathe in to prepare.

As you breathe out, peel your spine off the floor vertebra by vertebra. ① Finish in a C-curve (shoulders over hips, navel drawn back behind hips, and chin softly lowered towards the throat). ②

As you breathe in, straighten your spine.

Maintaining a straight spine, lean back approximately 15 degrees. ③

As you breathe out, lower your chin, softening it towards your chest, and curve your spine as you roll, vertebra by vertebra, back down to the floor.

Repetitions: Three.

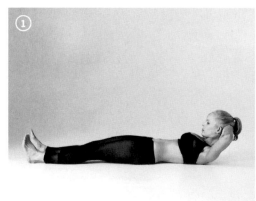
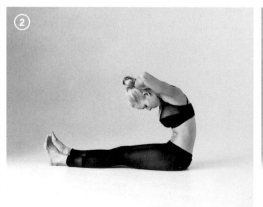
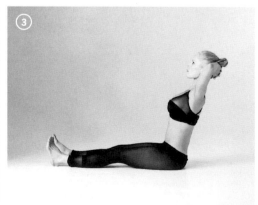

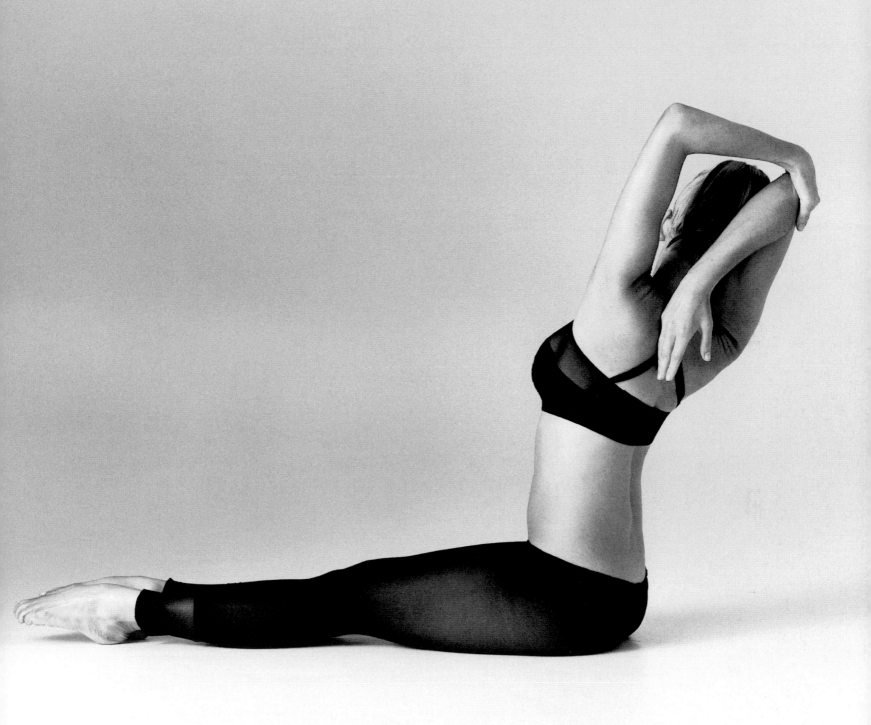

*Our mind and body are a continual work in progress. Enjoy the process;
our personal experiences lead us to our greatest achievements.*

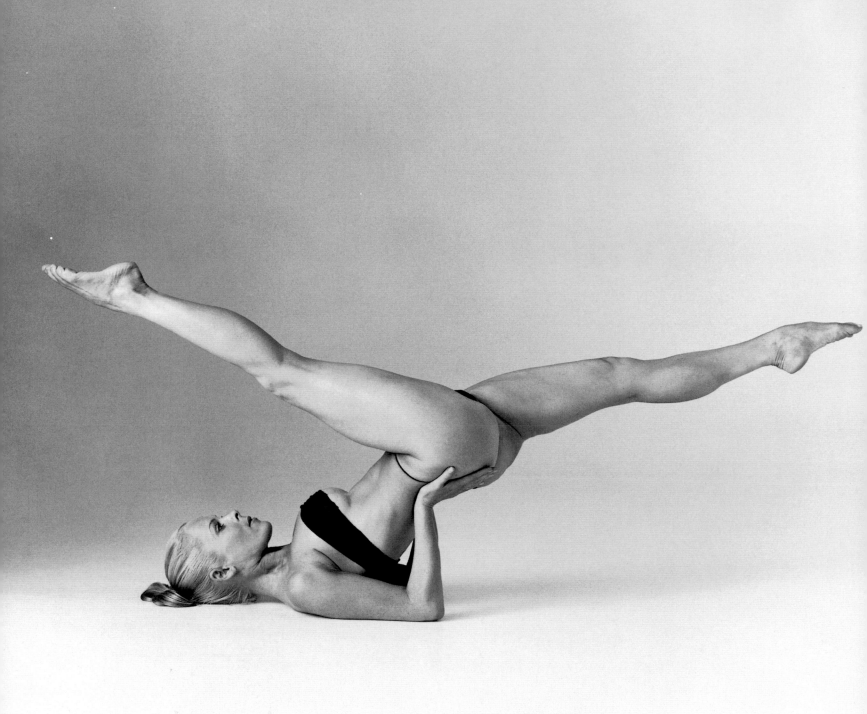

The highest form of control is learning when to release.

the scissors

focus Abdominals, pelvic stability and coordination.

imagery Visualise your legs crisscrossing like a pair of scissors.

precautions If you feel any discomfort in your neck, support your head with your hands or place your head on the floor. Stop if your lower back feels uncomfortable or weak.

point of interest Traditionally this exercise is followed by The Bicycle (see page 117); either flow the two exercises together or, if you are new to the exercises, separate them until you have mastered both.

tip The more slowly you do this exercise, the more control you will have over your pelvis.

Lie on your back, with your chest curled forward and your legs stretched straight up. Point your feet and stretch your arms out straight ahead at torso height, palms face-down. Anchor your tailbone and draw your navel firmly towards your spine, narrowing your waist.

Breathe in to prepare.

As you breathe out, simultaneously tighten the back of your left leg and extend it down until it

hovers just above the floor. Keep your pelvis strong and stable in its neutral position and keep your tailbone anchored to the floor. ①

As you breathe in, use a scissor motion to swap the position of your legs.

Repetitions: Five alternating to each side with your feet pointed and five to each side with your feet flexed.

》

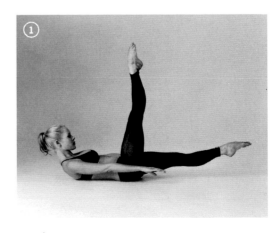

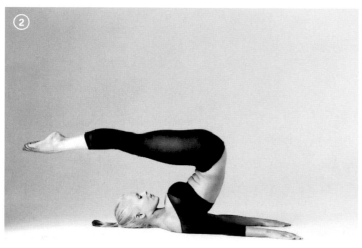

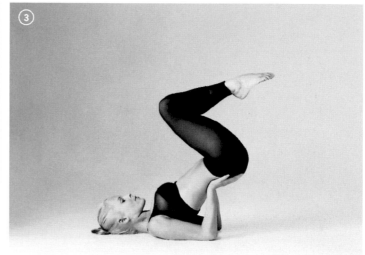

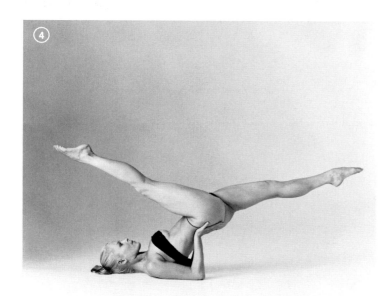

focus Balance, control and coordination.

imagery Visualise your pelvis sitting on a shelf and your legs moving like a pair of scissors.

precaution This exercise is inappropriate for people with a neck, shoulder or wrist issue. This exercise should be performed for the first time under experienced supervision.

Lie on your back, with your arms by your sides and your legs stretched straight up. Point your feet, anchor your tailbone and draw your navel firmly towards your spine, narrowing your waist.

Breathing naturally, use your abdominals to carry your legs over your head until they are parallel to the floor and your body weight is balanced between your shoulder blades. ②

Bend your knees and place the heels of your palms on your back at the top of your pelvis, with your fingertips pointing towards your tailbone. Allow your pelvis to lower into your palms as if it were sitting on a shelf. ③

Squeeze your inner thighs together, point your toes and stretch your legs in a straight line towards the ceiling.

Breathe in to prepare, holding your navel firmly towards your spine.

As you breathe out, use control to split your legs, sending your left leg forward and your right leg backward. Putting emphasis on your left leg, tighten the back of your thigh and match its depth with your right leg, to create a balanced V. ④

As you breathe in, use a scissor motion to swap the position of your legs.

Repetitions: Five each side.

Move straight on to The Bicycle (see page 117).

When confronted
with a challenge we
should consider our
greater goals and
appreciate every
small achievement
on the journey,
using the experience
to consolidate our
objectives.

the bicycle

focus Abdominals, pelvic stability and coordination.

imagery Visualise the motion of your legs as you ride a bicycle.

precaution If you feel any discomfort in your neck, support your head with your hands or place your head on the floor. Stop if your lower back feels uncomfortable or weak.

point of interest Traditionally this exercise continues straight on from The Scissors (see page 113); either flow the two exercises together or, if you are new to the exercises, separate them until you have mastered both.

tip The more slowly you do this exercise, the more control you will have over your pelvis.

Continuing on from the intermediate variation of The Scissors (see page 113) begin with your right leg stretched up towards the ceiling and your left leg stretched straight out a few inches off the floor. ① Breathe out as you visualise the motion your legs make as you ride a bicycle.

Bending your left leg, draw your heel towards your buttocks. ② Move your left thigh toward your chest as you stretch your right leg straight forward towards the floor.

As you breathe in, bend your right leg, drawing your heel towards your buttocks, then move your thigh towards your chest as you stretch your left leg straight forward towards the floor.

Repetitions: Five alternating to each side with your feet pointed and five to each side with your feet flexed.

»

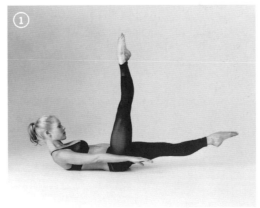

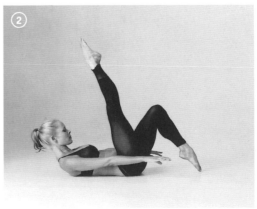

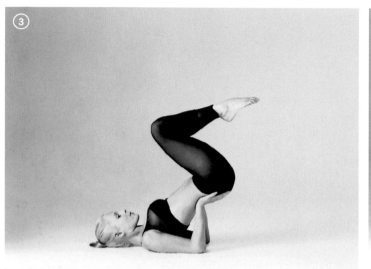

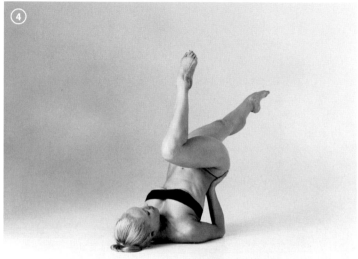

imagery Visualise your pelvis sitting on a shelf, and the motion your legs make as you ride a bicycle.

precaution It is inappropriate to attempt this exercise if you have a neck, shoulder or wrist issue. This exercise should be performed for the first time under experienced supervision.

Continuing on from the advanced–super-advanced variation of The Scissors (see page 115), visualise your pelvis sitting on a shelf. ③ Also visualise the motion your legs make as you ride a bicycle.

As you breathe out, bend your right leg, reaching your toes down towards the floor, trying to make contact with the floor while keeping your pelvis perfectly still. Draw your heel towards your buttocks as you fluidly continue to move your thigh toward your chest and stretch your left leg straight over your body and forward towards the floor. ④

As you breathe in, bend your left leg, reaching your toes down towards the floor, trying to make contact with the floor while keeping your pelvis perfectly still. Draw your heel towards your buttocks as you fluidly continue to move your thigh toward your chest and stretch your right leg straight over your body and forward towards the floor.

Repetitions: Five alternating to each side, and five alternating to each side reversing the bicycle.

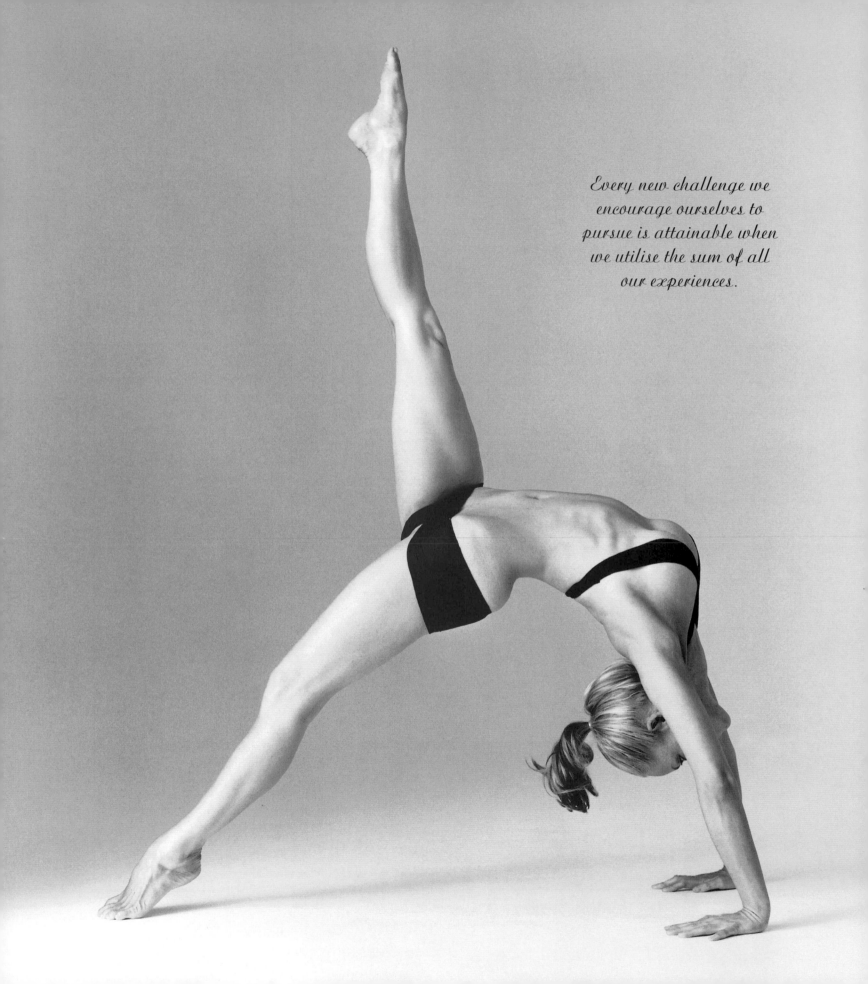

Every new challenge we encourage ourselves to pursue is attainable when we utilise the sum of all our experiences.

the shoulder bridge series

focus Spinal articulation, pelvic stability, the buttocks and the back of the thighs.

imagery Visualise your torso being completely still as your moving leg works freely, dissociating your pelvis from your thigh.

precaution Stop if you feel any lower-back or knee discomfort.

THE PELVIC ROLL-UP WITH TRANSFER

Lie on your back in a neutral-spine position, with your arms relaxed by your sides. Keeping your feet flat on the floor and hip-width apart, bend your legs up to a 90-degree angle at the knee joint, and make sure your ankles, knees and hips are in one line. Draw your navel down towards your spine and tighten your abdominals.

Breathe in to prepare.

As you breathe out, use your abdominals to press your lower back gently into the floor and lift your tailbone into the air, rolling each vertebra up from the floor one at a time and finishing with one long line between your knees, hips and shoulders. ①

Breathe in as you hold the position, maintaining a long neck, with your chin softly held in place.

As you breathe out, starting from your chest slowly lower each vertebra down to the floor one by one, like a string of pearls descending, finishing in the neutral-spine position.

Breathe in as you hold your neutral-spine position.

Repetitions: Two.

As you breathe out, use your abdominals to press your lower back gently into the floor and lift your tailbone into the air, rolling each vertebra up from the floor one at a time and finishing in one long line between your knees, hips and shoulders. ①

》

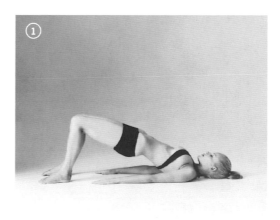

①

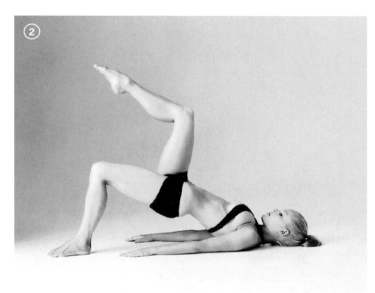

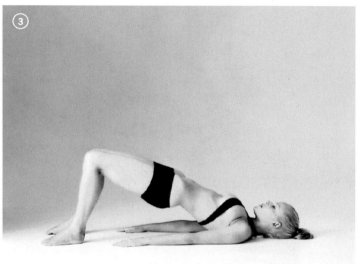

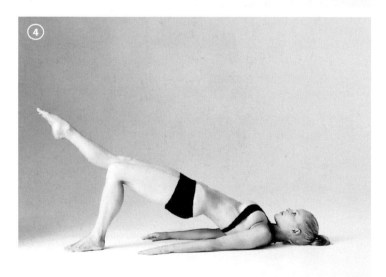

As you breathe in, tighten your left buttock and, keeping your hips very still, lift your right leg to a tabletop position (90 degrees at hip and knee). ②

As you breathe out, lower your right leg back down to the floor.

Repeat the process with your left leg.

Breathe in as you hold your hips still for a moment.

As you breathe out, starting from your chest slowly lower each vertebra down to the floor one by one, like a string of pearls descending, finishing in the neutral-spine position.

Breathe in as you hold your neutral-spine position.

Repetitions: Two sets.

Move on to The Hamstring Stretch (see page 125).

THE PELVIC ROLL-UP WITH LEG EXTENSION

Lie on your back in a neutral-spine position, with your arms relaxed by your sides. Keeping your feet flat on the floor and hip-width apart, bend your legs up to a 90-degree angle at the knee joint, and make sure your ankles, knees and hips are in one line. Draw your navel down towards your spine and tighten your abdominals.

Breathe in to prepare.

As you breathe out, use your abdominals to press your lower back gently into the floor and lift your tailbone into the air, rolling each vertebra off the floor one at a time and finishing in one long line between your knees, hips and shoulders. ③

As you breathe in, tighten your left buttock and, keeping your hips very still, lift your right leg to a tabletop position (90 degrees at hip and knee). ②

As you breathe out, straighten out your right leg with a pointed foot, finishing with both thighs on the same plane. ④

As you breathe in, return your right leg to the tabletop position.

As you breathe out, lower your right leg back down to the floor.

Repeat the process with your left leg.

As you breathe in, hold your hips still for a moment.

As you breathe out, starting from your chest slowly lower each vertebra down to the floor one by one, like a string of pearls descending, finishing in the neutral-spine position.

Breathe in as you hold your neutral-spine position.

Repetitions: Two sets.

Move on to The Hamstring Stretch (see page 125).

»

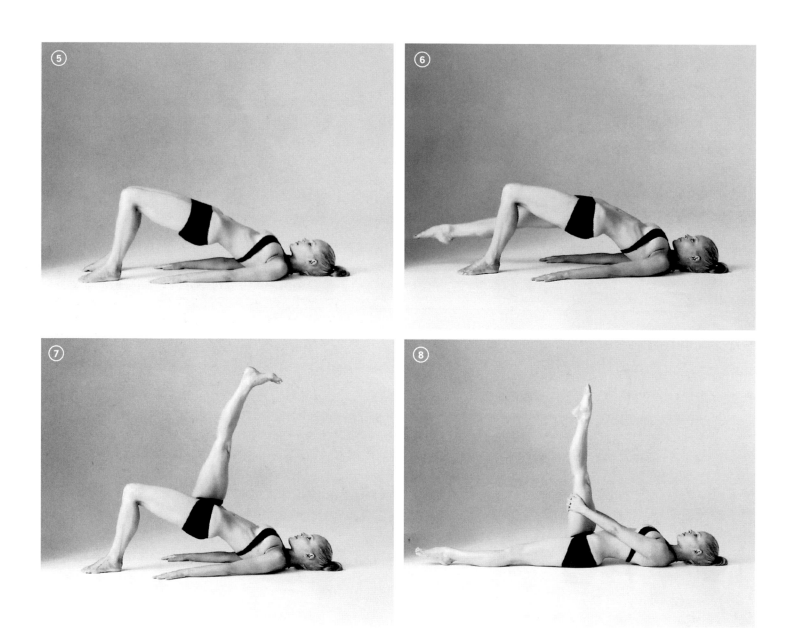

Lie on your back in a neutral-spine position, with your arms relaxed by your sides. Keeping your feet flat on the floor and hip-width apart, bend your legs up to a 90-degree angle at the knee joint, and make sure your ankles, knees and hips are in one line. Draw your navel down towards your spine and tighten your abdominals.

Breathe in to prepare.

As you breathe out, use your abdominals to press your lower back gently into the floor and lift your tailbone into the air, rolling each vertebra up from the floor one at a time and finishing in one long line between your knees, hips and shoulders. (5)

Breathe in as you hold the position, tightening your left buttock.

As you breathe out, point your right foot and slide it along the floor in front of you until your leg is straight. (6)

As you breathe in, flex your foot and lift your heel up towards the ceiling, maintaining a strong and stable pelvis. (7)

Maintaining a still pelvis, breathe out as you tighten the back of your right thigh, point your foot and reach it down and forward, as close to the floor as possible.

Repetitions: Ten.

Repeat the process with your left leg.

Keeping your hips lifted, breathe in as you return your left foot to the start position.

As you breathe out, soften your chest and roll each vertebra down to the floor one at a time, finishing in your neutral-spine position.

THE HAMSTRING STRETCH

focus To release the back of the thighs after the beginner and intermediate Shoulder Bridge Series.

precaution If you feel any lower-back discomfort during the stretch, bend the knee of your lower leg to release the restriction.

Lie on your back in a neutral-spine position. Reach your left leg out along the floor in front of you, pressing the back of your thigh firmly into the floor, keeping your heel anchored and your foot softly pointed. Stretch your right leg up into the air (if you feel tightness at the back of your thigh that restricts you achieving a vertical thigh and a neutral spine, bend your right knee a little) and hold onto the back of your right thigh with your hands, keeping your chin down and the back of your neck long. (8)

Draw your navel firmly towards your spine, narrowing your waist. Keeping your tailbone down and your spine in neutral to maximise the benefits of the stretch, pull your right leg carefully towards you until it has reached its limit. Flex your foot to increase the stretch further, lining your second and third toes up with the middle of your knee to maintain optimum alignment of your lower leg, and relax your chest, shoulders and neck.

Hold the stretch for six breaths; breathe slowly and naturally, drawing your navel firmly towards your spine.

Repetitions: One for each leg.

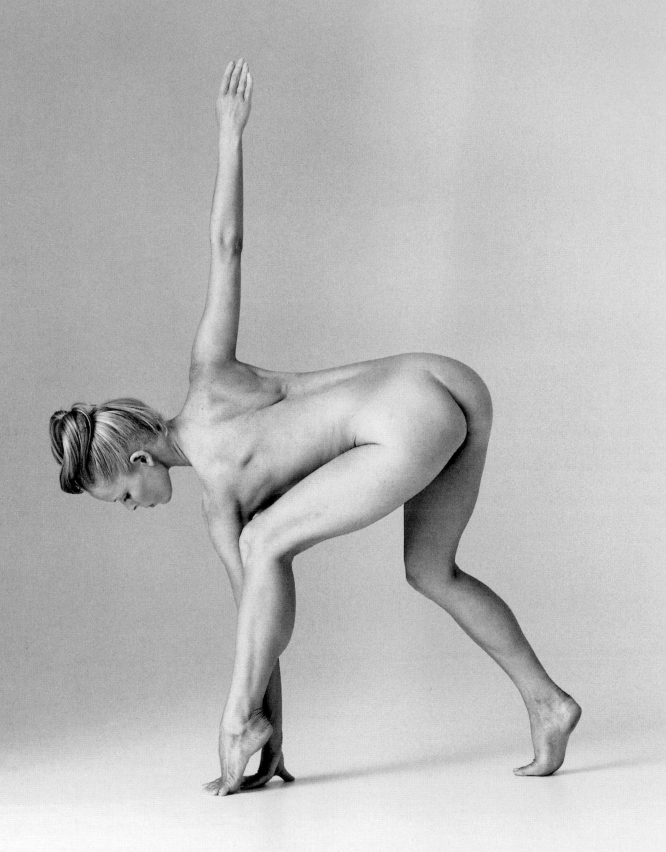

Enjoy the experience of learning every movement with precision and the subsequent ability to control your body and mind.

the spine twist

focus Spinal rotation, the seated posture (a co-contraction of the abdominals and spine extensors), abdominals and pelvic stability.

imagery As you are sitting tall, visualise the crown of your head reaching towards the ceiling and, as you move your body, that your torso and arms are sandwiched between two panes of glass.

precaution Stop if you feel any lower-back discomfort. If you feel any discomfort in your neck or shoulders, cross your arms over your chest and place your hands on your shoulders.

tip You need to sit very tall for this exercise. If you have difficulty getting your pelvis into a neutral position because your lower back, buttocks or legs are tight, sit on a rolled-up towel that is high enough for you to achieve the ideal position.

Sit tall, with your pelvis in neutral (hip bones and pubic bone on the same vertical plane) and your legs stretched out in front of you and squeezed together, feet flexed. Stretch your arms out to the sides of your body, parallel to the floor at chest height, palms face-down. Narrow your waist and lift your pelvic floor muscles, spiralling them up towards your ribs.

Breathe in to prepare.

Keeping your hips and ankles still, breathe out as you twist your body to the left, focusing on using your abdominals to rotate your spine. ①

To challenge your pelvic stability, add a small pulse and extra breath out (known as percussive breathing) to your torso. Visualise squeezing any remaining air out of your lungs and engaging your abdominals even further on your second breath out.

As you breathe in, return your torso and arms to centre.

Repetitions: Five alternating to each side.

Take your arms above your head, with your shoulders dropping down your back, palms facing each other.

Keeping your hips and ankles still, breathe out as you twist your body to the left, focusing on using your abdominals to rotate your spine, and adding a small pulse and percussive breath. ②

As you breathe in, return your torso and arms to centre.

Repetitions: Five alternating to each side. »

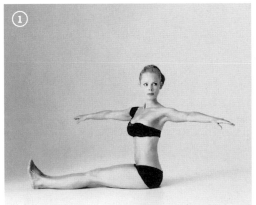

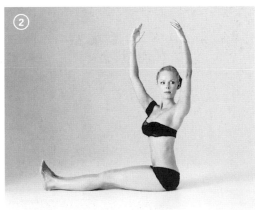

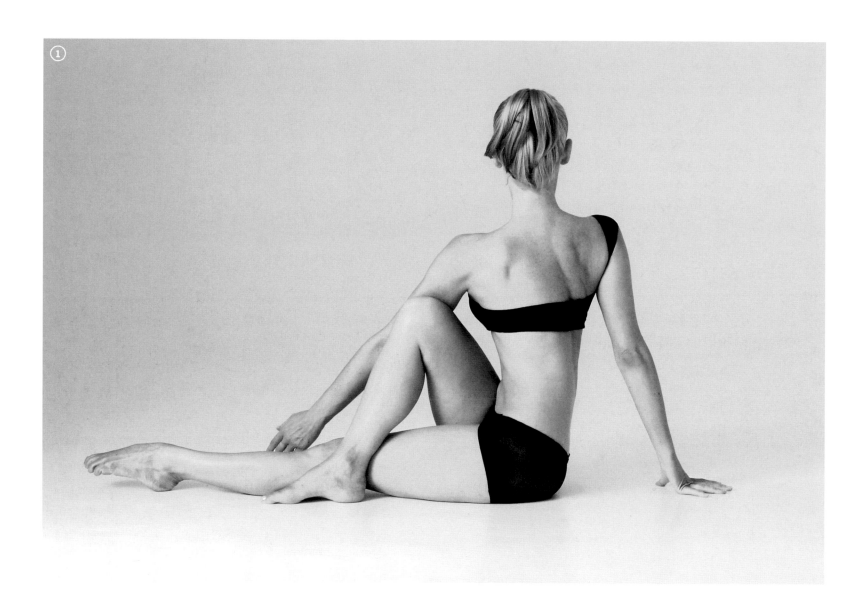

THE SPINE TWIST STRETCH

focus Spinal rotation stretch.

imagery As you are sitting tall, visualise the crown of your head reaching towards the ceiling and, as you move your body, that your torso and arms are sandwiched between two panes of glass.

precaution Stop if you feel any lower-back discomfort. If you feel any discomfort in your neck or shoulders, cross your arms over your chest and place your hands on your shoulders.

tip You need to sit very tall for this exercise, with your pelvis in neutral and your legs stretched out in front of you. If you have difficulty getting your pelvis into a neutral position because your lower back, buttocks or legs are tight, sit on a rolled-up towel that is high enough for you to achieve the ideal position.

   s

Sit tall, with your pelvis in neutral (hip bones and pubic bone on the same vertical plane) and your legs stretched out in front of you. Bend your right knee up and place your right foot on the floor to the left of your left knee.

Place your left arm in front of your right thigh and place your right hand on the floor behind you, pushing into the floor with the heel of your palm. ①

Anchor your sit bones and lengthen your spine towards the ceiling as you press your left arm and right leg against each other to facilitate the stretch of your spine and ribs.

Breathe in and out slowly and naturally six times as you hold the stretch.

Repetitions: One on each side.

the jackknife

focus Spinal articulation, control and balance.

imagery Visualise your hips moving like a smooth door hinge.

precaution Do not attempt this exercise if you have a neck, shoulder or lower-back issue.
This exercise should be performed for the first time under experienced supervision.

Lie on your back, with your arms by your sides. Lift your legs straight up, with a 90-degree angle at your hips. Point your feet and draw your navel to your spine, anchoring your tailbone. ①

Breathe in to prepare.

As you breathe out, focus on using your abdominals to carry your legs over your head until they are parallel to the floor and your body weight is balanced between your shoulder blades. ②

Keeping your legs straight, breathe in as you squeeze your buttocks and lift your legs straight up towards the ceiling, smoothly and carefully shifting your body weight onto the back of your shoulders. ③

As you breathe out, roll your spine, vertebra by vertebra, back down to the floor, keeping your legs stretched straight up. Visualise your toes being suspended from the ceiling and directly in line with your eyes on the descent, stretching out the back of your spine as you return to the start position.

As you breathe in, squeeze your buttocks and, keeping your legs straight, lower them down as close to the floor as possible without moving your lower back or pelvis. (The lower your legs, the more advanced the exercise.) Lift your legs back up to the start position.

Repetitions: Six.

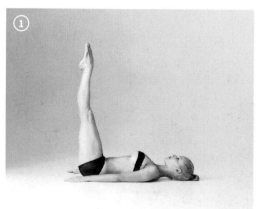

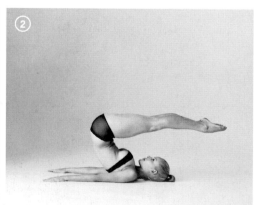

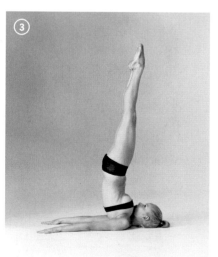

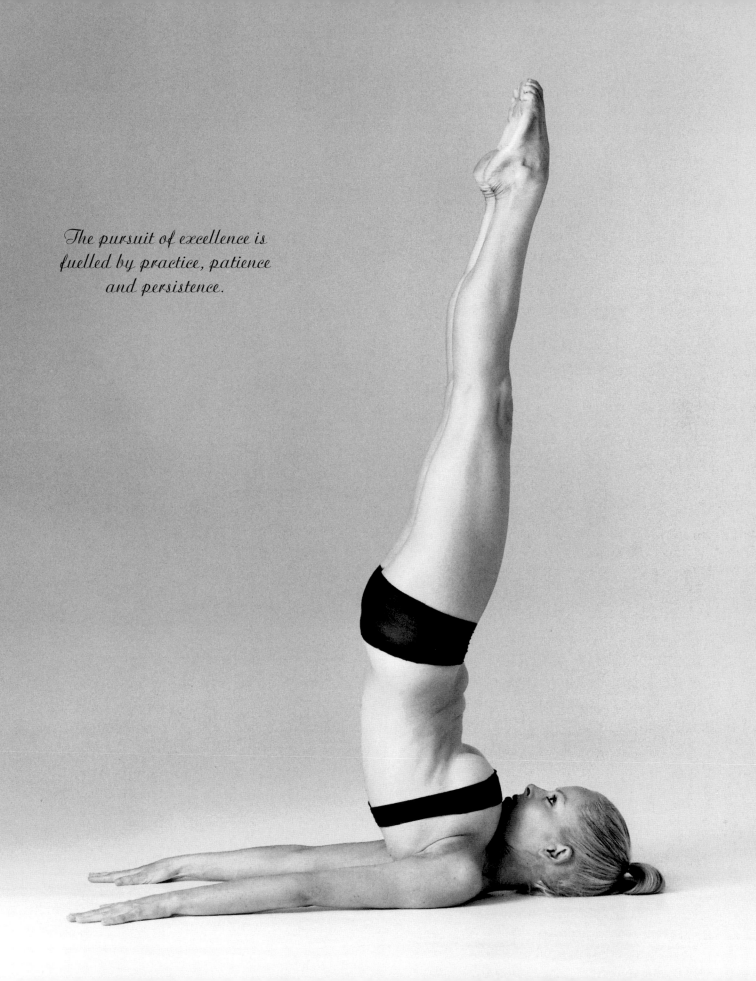

The pursuit of excellence is
fuelled by practice, patience
and persistence.

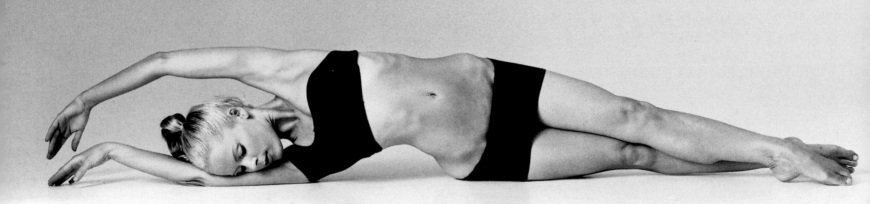

Solid foundations are the backbone of every new task we pursue. In our willingness to commence the journey, we undertake the responsibility to prepare our body for the future.

the side lifts

focus Lateral stabilisation, the sides of your abdominals, inner thighs, balance and control.

imagery Visualise lying on your side on a stretching rack and being pulled by your ankles, creating maximum length in your waist, hip joints and legs.

precaution Stop if you feel any lower-back discomfort. If you feel any shoulder discomfort, place a bigger cushion or towel underneath your head to support your neck, and place your underneath arm on the floor in front of your chest.

Lie on your right side, with your right arm stretched underneath you following the same alignment as your torso. Place a small cushion or rolled towel between your right ear and arm to support your neck and head. Place your left hand on the floor in front of you at chest height, with your shoulder and shoulder blade drawing down towards your hip, stabilising your shoulder girdle. Your shoulders and hips should be stacked one on top of the other, your toes pointed and your legs elongated and straight, a few inches in front of your body to assist in protecting your lower back.

Drawing your navel firmly towards your spine, lift your waist and ribs off the floor until you have a straight line that runs from the crown of your head, through the centre of your nose, sternum, navel and pubic bone (this is your neutral spine lying on your side). ①

Breathe in to prepare.

As you breathe out, lengthen both legs as far away from your hips as possible, and lift them a few inches off the floor, maintaining your neutral-spine position. ②

Keeping your legs squeezed together, breathe in as you lower both legs until they hover just above the floor.

Repetitions: Ten.

»

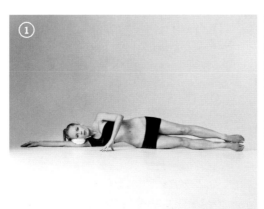
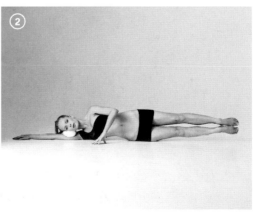

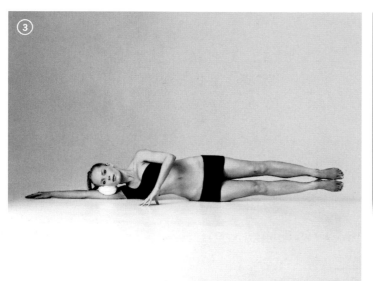

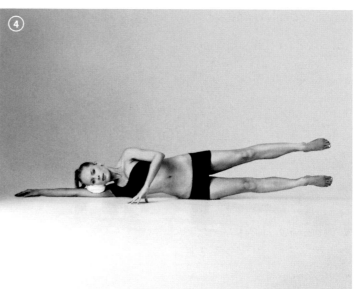

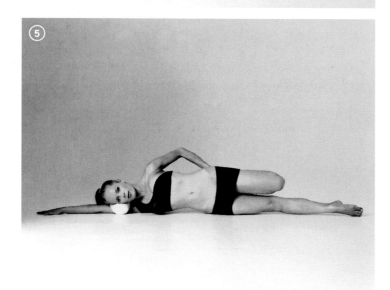

Hold your legs up after the last repetition as you breathe in. 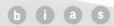③

As you breathe out, lift your upper leg a few inches towards the ceiling, using control to keep your hips still and stable and maintain your neutral spine. ④

As you breathe in, lower your upper leg, keeping your bottom leg lifted and strongly active. Neither leg should touch the floor.

Repetitions: Ten.

Breathe in, keeping your upper leg still and stable, as you lower your bottom leg until it hovers just above the floor.

As you breathe out, lift your bottom leg back up, using your inner thigh to squeeze your legs back together.

Repetitions: Ten.

variation ⓘ

When you have mastered the beginner variation of this exercise, challenge your balance and abdominals further by reaching your top arm straight up towards the ceiling as you perform the exercise. Ensure your top shoulder continues to press towards your hips, maintaining your shoulder-girdle stability.

Stay on the right side and continue The Side Kick Series (see page 137) before changing over to the left side.

variation ⓐ ⓢ

Challenge yourself further by increasing the tempo of the exercise.

Breathe in for the first repetition and breathe out for the second repetition, continuing in this manner until the exercise is completed.

Stay on the right side and continue The Side Kick Series (see page 137) before changing over to the left side.

THE QUAD STRETCH

focus To stretch out the front of your thighs.

precaution If you feel any discomfort in your knee, place a small towel or cushion behind the knee joint. Stop if the discomfort continues.

ⓑ ⓘ ⓐ ⓢ

Lie on your right side, with your right arm stretched underneath you following the same alignment as your torso. Place a small cushion or rolled towel between your right ear and arm to support your neck and head. Your shoulders and hips should be stacked one on top of the other and your legs elongated and straight, a few inches in front of your body to assist in protecting your lower back.

Breathing naturally, draw your navel firmly towards your spine, lifting your waist and ribs off the floor. Bend your left knee backwards and hold onto your left foot with your left hand. Keep your shoulders and shoulder blades drawn down towards your hip, stabilising your shoulder girdle, and keep your shoulders and hips stacked one on top of the other. Squeeze your left buttock, pushing it forward as you pull your knee back, facilitating the thigh stretch. ⑤

Repetitions: One on each side as you finish The Side Lifts.

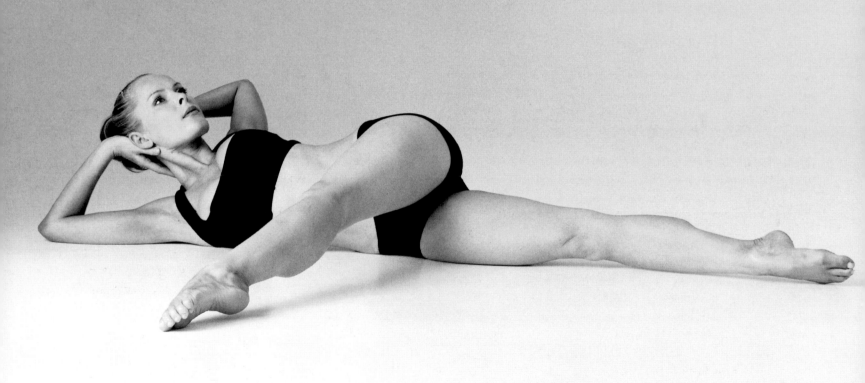

As you integrate your mind, body and spirit, you will learn to respect each aspect of your being and initiate movements intuitively from your heart.

the side kick series

focus Lateral stabilisation, balance, control, the sides of your abdominals and outer thighs.

imagery Visualise a sling wrapped underneath your waist holding up your torso.

precaution Stop if you feel any lower-back discomfort. If you feel any shoulder discomfort, lie on your side with your arm stretched underneath you following the same alignment as your torso. Place a small cushion or rolled towel between your ear and arm to support your neck and head. If you need to adapt the exercise even further, place a bigger pad underneath your head to support your neck, and place your lower arm on the floor in front of your chest.

variation I

Lie on your right side, propped up on your elbow, stretching your palm and forearm forward. Your elbow should be directly underneath your shoulder. Place your left hand on the floor in front of you at chest height, with your shoulders and shoulder blades drawing down towards your hips, stabilising your shoulder girdle. (To challenge your balance further, place your left hand behind your head throughout the exercise.)

Your hips should be stacked one on top of the other, your feet flexed and your legs straight and approximately 1 foot forward from your body. Push firmly into your right elbow, imagining a sling lifting your waist upwards until there is one long incline from your pelvis to your head, then draw your navel towards your spine to stabilise your torso. Keeping your legs straight, lift your left leg to hip height.

As you breathe in, swing your left leg forward, still at hip height, as far as you can while maintaining a stable and still torso and keeping your foot flexed. ①

As you breathe out, squeeze your buttocks, point your left foot and swing your left leg back as far as you can, keeping your torso still.

Repetitions: Ten sets on each side.

Start with your right elbow on a diagonal away from your shoulder and your right hand behind your head. Your body should now be significantly closer to the floor but still lifted under your torso by your imaginary sling. Place your left hand behind your head.

As you breathe in, swing your left leg forward as far as you can, pulsing your leg once. This quick movement challenges your torso's stability and balance.

As you breathe out, squeeze your left buttock and point your foot as you swing your leg backward, once again adding the pulse and keeping your torso still.

Repetitions: Ten sets on each side.

Focus on maintaining a stable torso, and allow your top leg to swing independently, dissociating your thigh from your pelvis. »

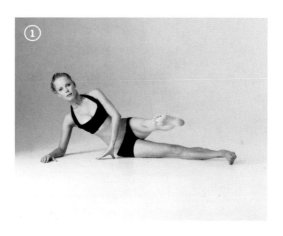

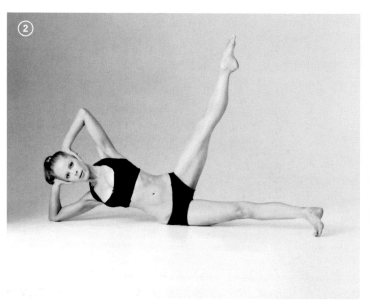

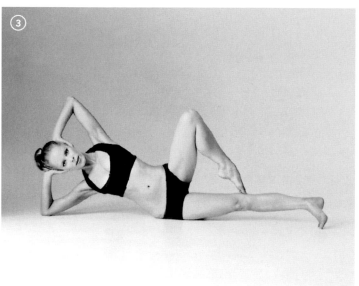

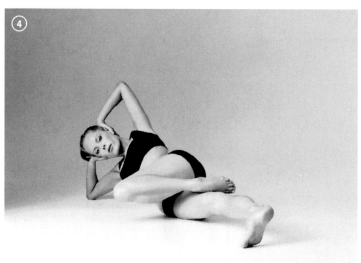

variation

There are many advanced variations in The Side Kick Series. Here are four of them.

variation II up/down

As you breathe in, swing your left leg straight up towards the ceiling, with your foot pointed and your thigh turned out as far as possible, keeping your torso completely still. ②

As you breathe out, flex your foot and return your leg to the start position, maintaining the turn-out in your thigh.

Repetitions: Five leading with a pointed foot and five leading with a flexed foot.

variation III developes

As you breathe in, bend your left knee, sliding your toes up towards your right knee. ③

Lift and straighten your left leg toward the ceiling, with your foot pointed and your thigh turned out, keeping your torso completely still. ②

As you breathe out, flex your foot and return the straight leg to the start position, maintaining the turn-out of your thigh.

Repetitions: Five.

As you breathe in, flex your left foot, lifting your left leg toward the ceiling, with the leg turned out, keeping your torso completely still.

As you breathe out, point your left foot and, bending your left knee, place the toes of your left foot on your right knee. Slide your toes down towards your ankle, returning the leg to the start position.

Repetitions: Five.

variation IV the bicycle

As you breathe in, swing your left leg forward as far as you can, with your left foot flexed and your torso still. Bend your left heel in towards your buttocks, pointing your left foot. ④

As you breathe out, keep your heel squeezed in close to your buttocks and carry your left knee back behind your hips, stretching out the front of your hip and thigh. Extend and straighten your left leg straight behind your body, maintaining a still torso. Return to the start position.

Repetitions: Five initiating forward and five initiating back.

variation V big circles

As you breathe in, swing your left leg forward as far as you can, with your left foot pointed, your leg turned out and your torso still, then continue carrying your leg straight up towards the ceiling.

As you breathe out, hold your torso still as you carry your left leg behind you, then complete the circle by returning your left leg to the start position.

Repetitions: Five in each direction.

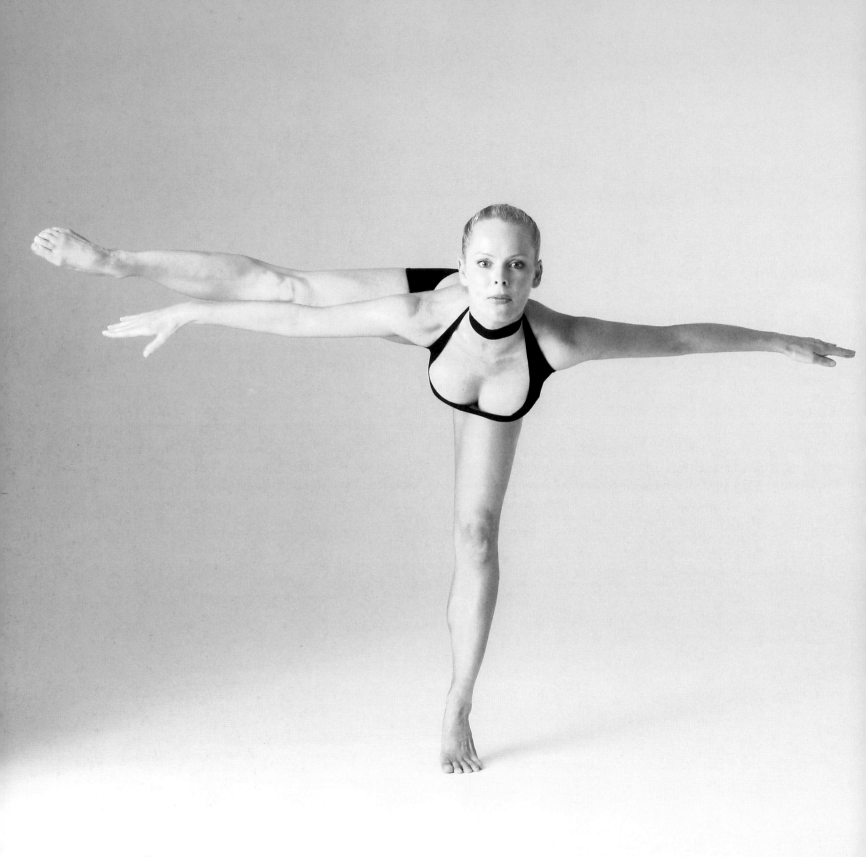

Creation begins with an inspired action.

the leg lifts

focus To give you that famous Pilates butt!

imagery As you are lying on your side, visualise your neutral spine position against a wall as you move the working leg independently, dissociating your thighs from your pelvis.

precaution Stop if you feel any lower-back discomfort. If you feel any shoulder discomfort, place a bigger pad underneath your head to support your neck, and place your arm on the floor in front of your chest.

tip This is one of those 'feel the burn' exercises. The more slowly and controlled you make each movement, the more intense it will be.

Lie on your right side with your right arm stretched underneath you following the same alignment as your torso. Place a small cushion or rolled towel between your right ear and arm to support your neck and head. Place your left hand on the floor in front of you at chest height, with your shoulders and shoulder blades drawing down towards your hips, stabilising your shoulder girdle. Your shoulders and hips should be stacked one on top of the other, and your left leg elongated and straight in a line that follows your body. Bend your right leg up underneath you until you have a 90-degree angle at the hip and knee.

Flex your left foot and rotate it so your heel faces up towards the ceiling and your toes point down towards the floor.

Drawing your navel firmly towards your spine, lift your waist and ribs off the floor until you have a straight spine and a line that runs from the crown of your head, through the centre of your nose, sternum, navel and pubic bone (this is your neutral spine lying on your side).

Breathe in to prepare.

As you breathe out, reach your left heel as far away from your hip as possible and lift it a few inches, keeping your hip and torso stable. ①

As you breathe in, lower your leg, keeping your toes just off the floor.

Repetitions: Ten. »

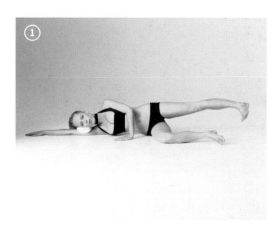

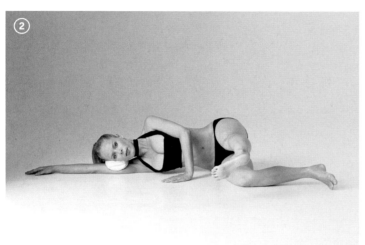

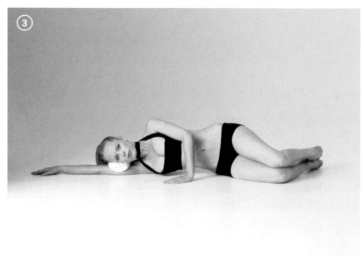

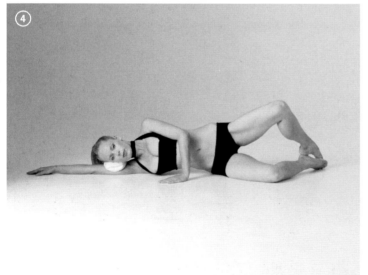

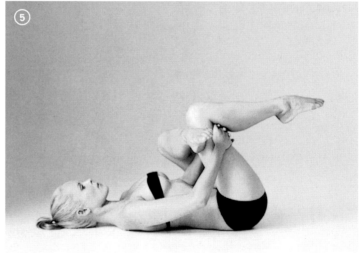

As you breathe out, carry your left leg forward towards your navel, maintaining your neutral spine.

Leading with your heel, lift your leg a few inches.

As you breathe in, lower your leg and return to the start position.

Repetitions: Ten.

As you breathe out, carry your left leg forward towards your navel, maintaining your neutral spine.

Leading with your heel, lift your leg a few inches.

As you breathe in, lower your leg until your toes hover just above the floor.

As you breathe out, lift your leg a few inches, leading with your heel.

Repetitions: Ten.

Place your left leg on top of the right in the tabletop position (90 degrees at hip and knee). Slide your feet back until they line up with your hip joints, maintaining the 90-degree angle at your knees.

Place your left hand at the back of your left buttock to assist in keeping your hips still. When you are satisfied that you have mastered the technique of keeping your pelvis still, place your left hand on the floor in front of you at chest height.

Breathe in to prepare.

Keeping your feet on the floor and your hips still, breathe out as you lift your left knee as high as possible.

As you breathe in, lower your left leg back down.

Repetitions: Ten.

variation **a** **s**

As you carry your leg forward in the second phase of the exercise, add an extra heel lift to each repetition – on the second repetition lift twice, on the third repetition lift three times . . . until you have reached ten.

When you are satisfied that you have mastered the art of keeping your hips still, challenge your balance and abdominals further by placing your left hand behind your head with your elbow reaching up towards the ceiling as you perform the exercise.

THE BUTTOCK STRETCH

b **i** **a** **s**

focus To stretch the buttocks.

precaution Stop if you feel any lower-back or knee discomfort. If you have difficulty keeping the back of your head on the floor, place a towel or cushion underneath your head.

Lie on your back, with your arms relaxed by your sides. Keeping your feet flat on the floor and slightly apart, bend your legs up to a 90-degree angle at the knee joint. Lifting your left leg up, place your left ankle over your right knee and open your left knee out to the side.

Reach both hands behind your right thigh and clasp them together. Lift your knees towards your chest, keeping your left knee open. To maximise the effectiveness of this stretch, focus on keeping your tailbone anchored to the floor as you hug your knees close to your chest, dissociating your thighs from your pelvis.

Breathe in and out slowly and naturally six times as you hold the stretch.

Repeat with your right knee open.

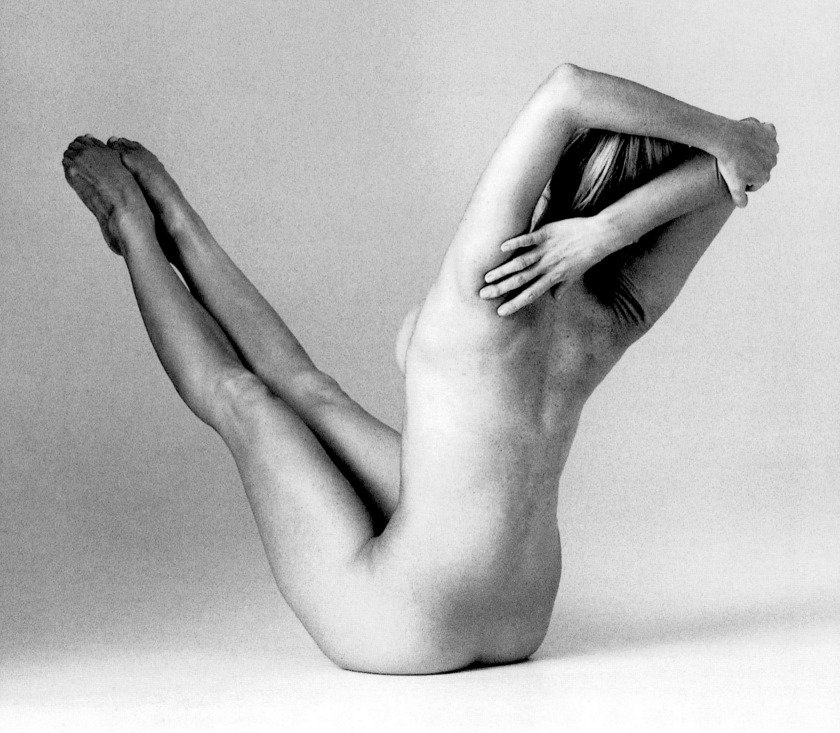

Every challenge we fulfil has a tremendous impact on our future achievements.

the teaser

focus Abdominals, hip flexors, spinal articulation, balance and control.

imagery Visualise your body in a perfect letter V, with your eye-line and toes remaining on the same plane as you move.

precaution Stop if you feel any discomfort in your lower back.

prerequisite You need to be strong and competent at The Roll-up (see page 59) before attempting this exercise.

PREPARATION I

Sit tall with your back straight, shoulders over hips, legs in front of your body, feet flat on the floor and knees bent. Hold on underneath your thighs, draw your navel towards your spine and keep your abdominals tight. Maintaining a straight back, lean back to create the letter V with your body. Keeping the insides of your knees together, stretch your right leg out in front of you, with your toes pointed and your upper thighs aligned on the same plane. ①

Breathe in to prepare.

As you breathe out, gently lower your chin, soften your chest and use your abdominals to curve your navel behind your hips as you tuck your pelvis. Use control to walk your hands down the backs of your thighs as you roll each vertebra down one at a time. ② Finish by lengthening your entire spine along the floor. ③

Breathe in and hold the position.

As you breathe out, lengthen the crown of your head behind you, allowing your chin to soften slightly towards your chest as you deepen into your abdominals and peel each vertebra off the floor, finishing in the V position with your shoulders down and your chest open.

Repetitions: Two before changing to the left leg.

When you have mastered all aspects of this exercise you are ready to continue on to the next progression. »

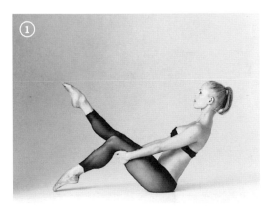 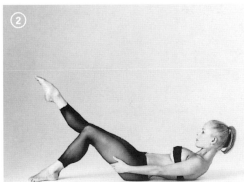 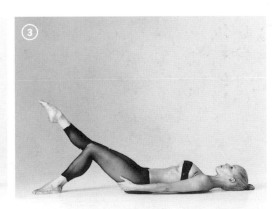

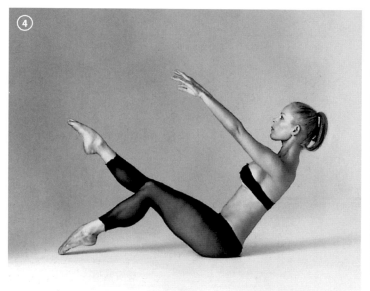

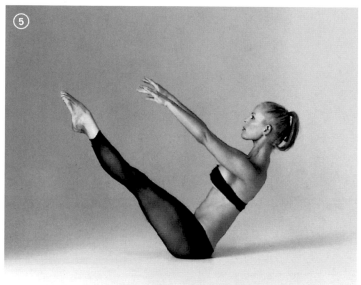

PREPARATION II

Start in your V position, with your right leg elongated off the floor in front of you. Stretch your arms up on an incline that runs parallel to your right leg. ④

Breathe in to prepare, drawing your navel firmly towards your spine.

As you breathe out, gently lower your chin, soften your chest and use your abdominals to curve your navel back behind your hips, tucking your pelvis as you slowly descend your spine, vertebra by vertebra, towards the floor. As you lower your body towards the floor, allow your arms to fluidly follow the line of your legs and then reach straight over your head as the base of your shoulder comes into contact with the floor, and continue on to the floor behind you as the remainder of your spine elongates along the floor.

Breathe in and hold the position.

As you breathe out, lengthen the crown of your head behind you, allowing your chin to soften slightly towards your chest as you deepen into your abdominals and peel each vertebra off the floor, floating your arms over your head and returning them to their start position as your torso returns to its start position, with your shoulders down and your chest open.

Repetitions: Two before changing to the left leg.

When you have mastered all aspects of this exercise you are ready to continue on to the next progression.

TEASER I

tip To make the exercise a little easier, hold onto the back of your thighs and walk your hands slowly down then up.

Start balanced in your V position, with both legs elongated off the floor in front of you and your toes pointed. Stretch your arms up on an incline that runs parallel to your legs, with your palms face-down and your fingertips lengthening away from your shoulders. Draw your navel firmly towards your spine. ⑤

Breathe in to prepare.

As you breathe out, gently lower your chin, soften your chest and use your abdominals to curve your navel back behind your hips, tucking your pelvis as you slowly descend your spine, vertebra by vertebra, towards the floor. As you lower your body towards the floor, allow your arms to fluidly follow the line of your legs and then reach straight over your head as the base of your shoulder comes into contact with the floor, and continue on to the floor behind you as the remainder of your spine elongates along the floor.

Breathe in and hold the position.

As you breathe out, lengthen the crown of your head behind you, allowing your chin to soften slightly towards your chest as you deepen into your abdominals and peel each vertebra off the floor, floating your arms over your head and allowing them to return to their start position as your torso returns to its start position, with your shoulders down and your chest open.

Repetitions: Four.

When you have mastered all aspects of this exercise you are ready to continue on to the next progression.

»

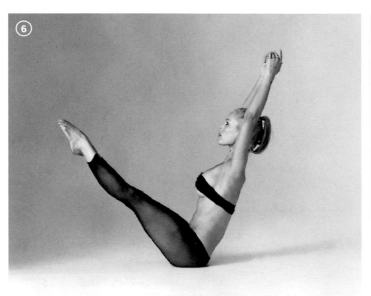

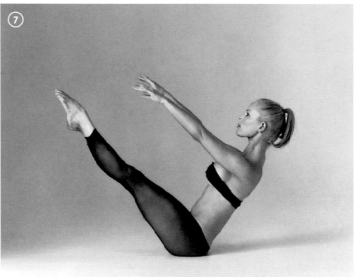

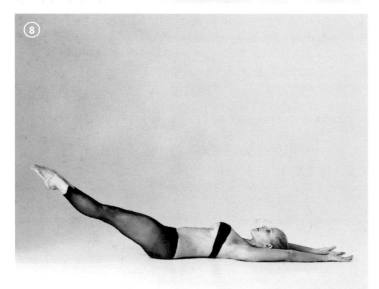

TEASER II

Start balanced in your V position, with both legs elongated off the floor in front of you and your toes pointed. Stretch your arms up beside your ears, with palms facing each other and fingertips lengthening away from your shoulders. Press your shoulders down your back and towards your hips, and draw your navel firmly towards your spine. ⑥

Breathe in to prepare.

Keeping your torso and arms still, breathe out as you lower your legs as close to the floor as possible.

As you breathe in, return to the start position.

Repetitions: Four.

When you have mastered all aspects of this exercise you are ready to continue on to the next progression.

TEASER III

Start balanced in your V position, with both legs elongated off the floor in front of you and your toes pointed. Stretch your arms up on an incline that runs parallel to your legs, with your palms face-down and your fingertips lengthening away from your shoulders. Draw your navel firmly towards your spine. ⑦

Breathe in to prepare.

As you breathe out, gently lower your chin, soften your chest and use your abdominals to curve your navel back behind your hips, tucking your pelvis as you slowly lower both legs and descend your spine, vertebra by vertebra, towards the floor. As you lower your body and legs towards the floor, keep your eye-line on your toes and allow your arms to fluidly follow the line of your legs and then reach straight over your head as the base of your shoulder comes into contact with the floor, and continue on to the floor behind you as the remainder of your spine elongates along the floor. Stop your legs lowering at this point so that they hover just off the floor. ⑧

Breathe in and hold the position.

As you breathe out, keeping your eye-line on your toes, lengthen the crown of your head behind you, allowing your chin to soften slightly towards your chest as you deepen into your abdominals and peel each vertebra off the floor, floating your arms over your head and allowing them to return to their start position as your torso returns to its start position, with your shoulders down and your chest open.

Repetitions: Four.

hip circles

focus Abdominals, hip flexors, balance, control and coordination.

imagery Visualise your legs drawing a perfect circle in the air in front of you.

precaution If you feel any lower-back discomfort, stop the exercise. To simplify and make the exercise easier while you are developing your skill and endurance, prop yourself up on your elbows, pressing them strongly into the floor to keep your neck and shoulders high and strong.

Sit tall with your back straight, shoulders over hips, legs in front of your body, feet flat on the floor and knees bent. Hold on underneath your thighs, draw your navel towards your spine and keep your abdominals tight. Maintaining a straight back, lean back to create the letter V with your body. Place your hands palm-down approximately 2 feet behind you, with your fingertips facing away from your body, and lift your legs up to form a V with your body. Allow your arms to comfortably support the posture of your body. ①

Breathe in to prepare.

As you breathe out, squeeze your legs together and circle them towards the right and down towards the floor.

As you breathe in, complete the circle and finish in the start position.

Repetitions: Four alternating in each direction.

Start balanced in your V position, with both legs elongated off the floor in front of you and your toes pointed. Stretch both arms up on an incline that runs parallel to your legs, with your palms face-down and your fingertips lengthening away from your shoulders. Draw your navel firmly towards your spine.

Breathe in to prepare.

As you breathe out, squeeze your legs together and circle them towards the right and down towards the floor as both arms circle towards the left and up towards the ceiling.

As you breathe in, complete the leg and arm circles and finish in the start position.

Repetitions: Four alternating in each direction.

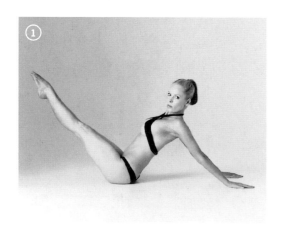

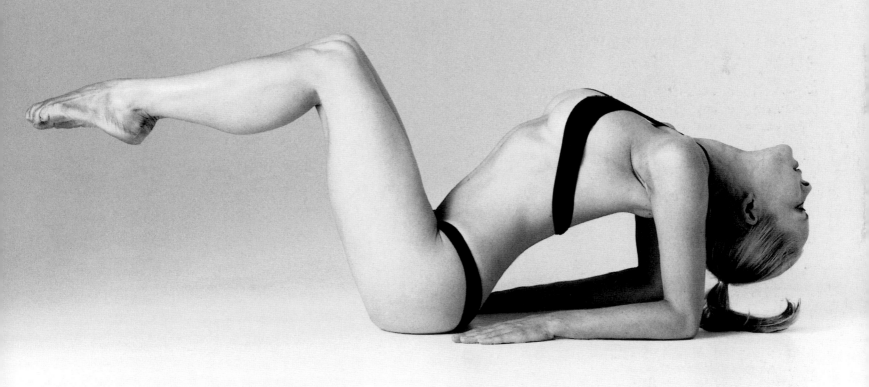

Concentration is a vital key to control. Remember, if your mind wanders from its purpose, your body will follow.

the cancan

focus To release the spine after The Teaser and The Hip Circles.

imagery A little Cancan at the Moulin Rouge!

precaution Stop if you feel any lower-back discomfort.

Sit tall with your back straight, shoulders over hips, legs in front of your body, knees bent, feet pointed and the tips of your toes touching the floor. Keeping your back straight, lean back to create the letter V with your body. Place your hands palm-down approximately 2 feet behind you, with your fingertips facing away from your body. Allow your arms to comfortably support the posture of your body. Draw your navel firmly towards your spine, tightening your abdominals.

As you breathe in, turn your head to the right and gracefully lower both knees to the left, indulging in the stretch and release of your torso. ①

As you breathe out, turn your head to the left and gracefully lower both knees over to the right, once again indulging in the stretch and release of your torso.

As you breathe in, turn your head to the right and gracefully lower both knees over to the left.

As you breathe out, straighten your legs into a V position, holding the pose momentarily. ② Bend your legs and return the tips of your toes to the floor.

Repetitions: Two alternating to each side.

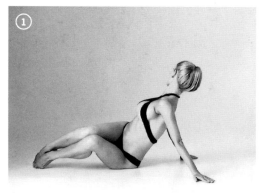

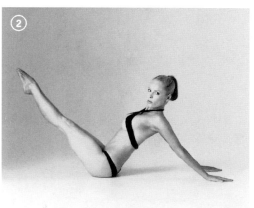

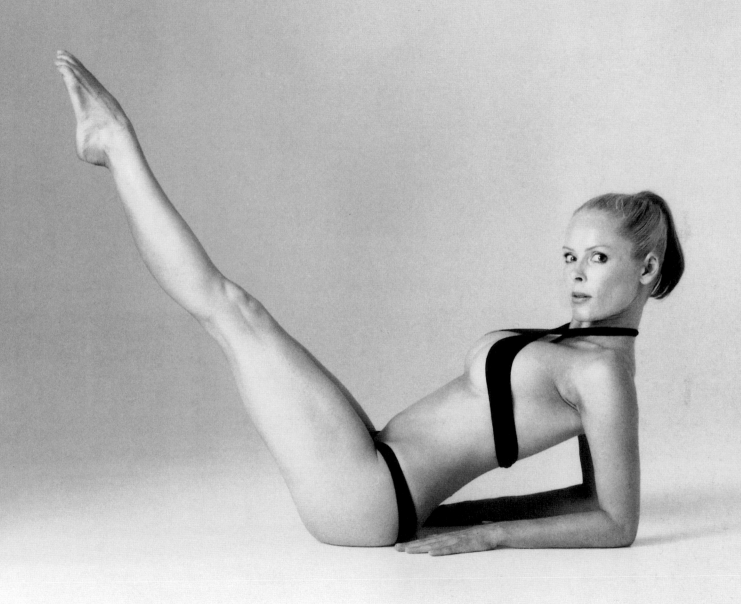

By opening our heart we rejuvenate our body.

swimming

focus Spine extension and coordination.

imagery Visualise yourself balancing your torso with control on the peak of a rounded mound as your arms and legs flutter independently.

precaution If you feel any lower-back discomfort, stop the exercise and move into The Rest Position (see page 108) to release your lower back. If you experience any shoulder discomfort, rest your arms on the floor beside your body, eliminating them from the exercise.

b

Lie face-down, with your forehead resting on a small cushion or rolled towel, allowing room for your nose so you can breathe freely. Stretch your arms out in front of you on the floor, with your palms face-down, and draw your shoulders down your back and away from your ears. Gently move your pubic bone down towards the floor until it rests on the same plane as the front of your hips (this is your neutral pelvis). Lengthen your legs to hip width along the floor behind you, with the backs of your knees and the soles of your feet facing the ceiling, and your feet pointed. Drawing your navel firmly towards your spine, tighten your abdominals and lower buttock muscles to assist in maintaining a strong and stable pelvis.

Breathe in to prepare.

As you breathe out, lift your right arm and left leg a few inches off the floor, taking care to keep your right shoulder away from your ear, and the front of your left hip and pubic bone firmly anchored into the floor, with your lower buttocks maintaining a stable pelvis. ①

As you breathe in, return to the start position.

Repetitions: Five alternating to each side.

variation **i**

To make this exercise a little more challenging, as you lift your right arm and left leg, also lift your chest, extending your spine and lengthening the crown of your head forward, your chin softly tucked towards your throat and your eye-line down. ②

Repetitions: Five alternating to each side.

variation **a** **s**

Continuing on from the intermediate variation, lift your chest into spinal extension as both arms and legs lift a few inches off the floor. ③

As you breathe in, alternate the basic swimming action four times.

As you breathe out, alternate the basic swimming action four times.

Repetitions: Five complete breaths.

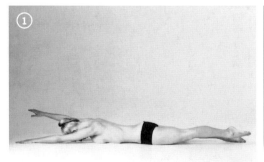

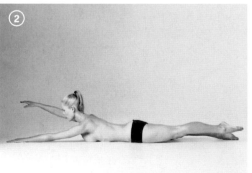

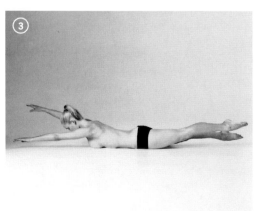

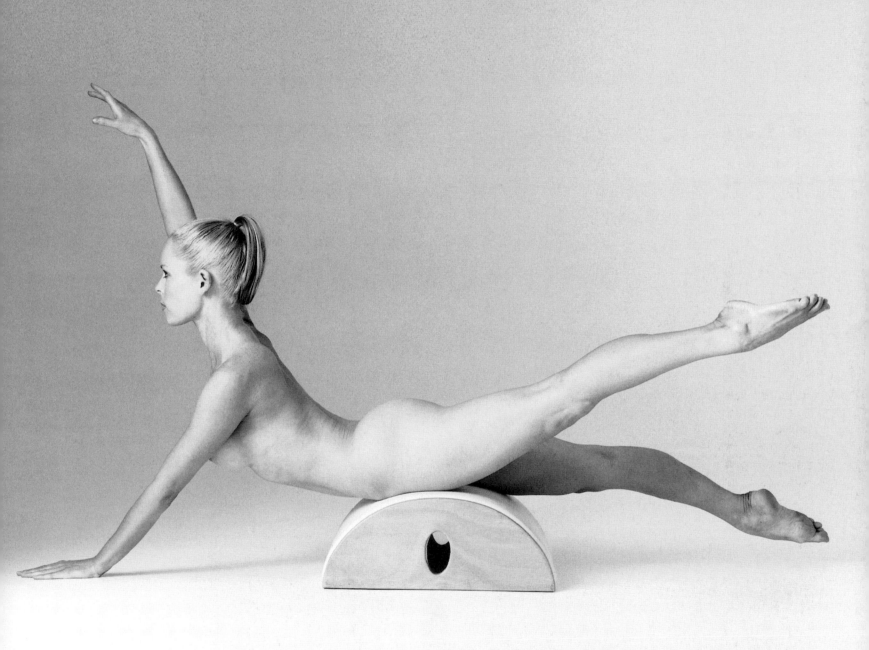

Graceful movement is the poetry of the body.

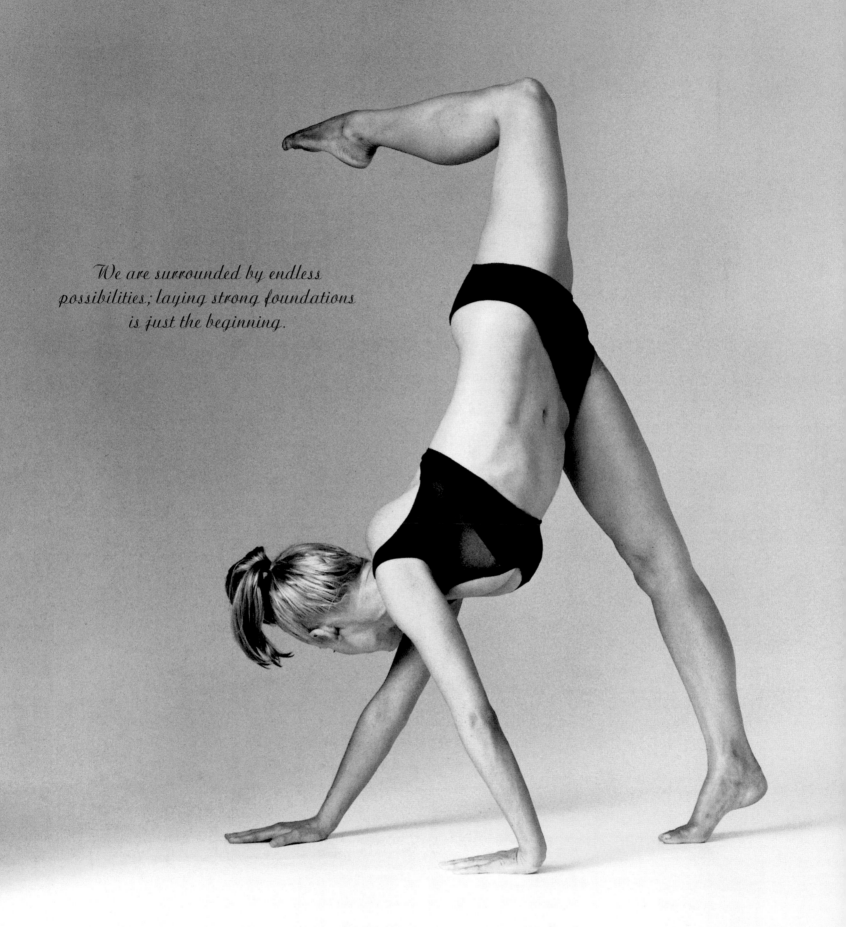

We are surrounded by endless possibilities; laying strong foundations is just the beginning.

the up-stretch

focus Core conditioning, strengthening the upper back and chest, and stretching the hamstrings and calves.

imagery Visualise your body in pyramid and plank positions.

precaution Stop if you feel any lower-back, shoulder or wrist discomfort.

b **i**

Sit back on your heels, with your knees and ankles slightly apart and your toes lifted underneath you so you are on the balls of your feet. Lay your chest forward over your thighs, and stretch both arms out on the floor in front of your body, with the palms of your hands pressing firmly into the floor a little wider than your shoulders. Relax the crown of your head towards the floor. ①

Breathe in to prepare.

As you breathe out, lift your pelvis into the air to form a pyramid with your body, pressing your heels down towards the floor and stretching out the back of your calves and thighs. ②

Breathing naturally, draw both shoulders down your back towards your hips and gently turn your head from side to side to release any tension in your neck. You should have a straight line running up from the heels of your palms to your tailbone, and a straight line from your tailbone down to the heels of your feet.

Breathe in and hold this position.

Keeping your heels as low as possible, breathe out as you transfer your body forward into a plank position, with one long line from the crown of your head to your heels. Your shoulders should be directly over your wrists. To align your neck, visualise the heels of your palms as the base of a triangle and your eye-line as the pinnacle of that triangle. ③ »

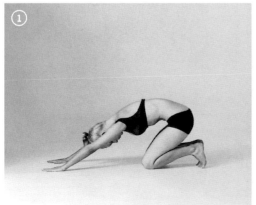

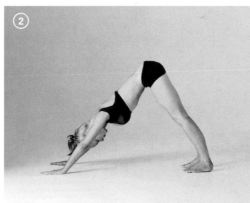

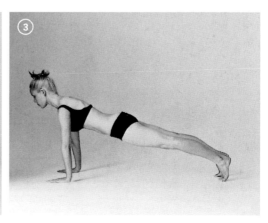

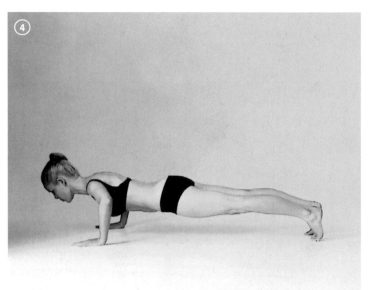

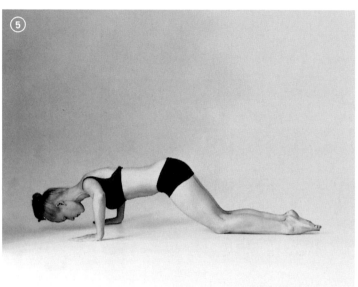

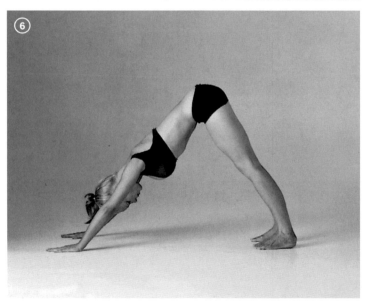

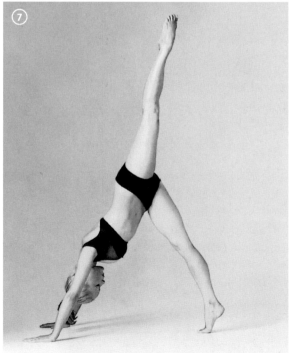

Breathe in and hold the position, keeping your navel drawn firmly towards your spine.

As you breathe out, return to the pyramid position.

Repetitions: Five.

Breathe in and hold this position.

As you breathe out, transfer your body into a plank position.

Keeping your shoulder blades apart, breathe in as you bend your elbows out to your sides, keeping your neck long and your torso stable as you lower your body as far as you can while maintaining control. ④ To decrease the intensity of the push-ups, lower your knees to the floor in the plank position while keeping your tailbone lifted. ⑤

As you breathe out, straighten your arms, maintaining a strong and stable plank position.

Repetitions: Ten.

As you breathe in, lower your knees gently to the floor.

As you breathe out, sit back on your heels, releasing the balls of your feet and allowing the top of your instep to rest on the floor.

Sit back on your heels, with your knees and ankles slightly apart and your toes lifted underneath you so you are on the balls of your feet. Lay your chest forward over your thighs, and stretch both arms out on the floor in front of your body, with the palms of your hands pressing firmly into the floor a little wider than your shoulders. Relax the crown of your head towards the floor.

Breathe in to prepare.

As you breathe out, lift your pelvis into the air, pressing your heels down towards the floor, stretching out the back of your calves and thighs. ⑥

Breathing naturally, draw both shoulders down your back towards your hips, and gently turn your head from side to side to release any tension in your neck. You should have a straight line running up from the heels of your palms to your tailbone, and a straight line from your tailbone down to the heels of your feet.

Breathe in and hold this position.

As you breathe out, point your left foot and lift your leg as high into the air as you can, keeping your hips square and your thighs straight. ⑦

Breathe in and hold this position.

Keeping your right heel as low as possible, breathe out as you transfer your body into a plank position, keeping your left leg lengthened behind you and raised a few inches off the floor. Your shoulders should be directly over your wrists. To align your neck, visualise the heels of your palms as the base of a triangle and your eye-line as the pinnacle of that triangle.

Breathe in and hold this position, keeping your navel drawn firmly towards your spine.

As you breathe out, return to the split position.

Repetitions: Five.

Keeping your right heel as low as possible, breathe in as you bend your elbows out to your sides, stretching the crown of your head diagonally down towards the floor and keeping your left leg lengthened up behind you in a split.

As you breathe out, straighten your arms.

Repetitions: Five.

As you breathe in, place your left leg down, returning to the pyramid position.

Repeat with your right leg lifted in a split.

the leg pull front

focus Torso stabilisation and upper-body strength.

imagery Visualise your body in a plank position, with one long line from the crown of your head to your heels.

precaution If you feel any discomfort in your lower back, place your knees on the floor. If you feel any discomfort in your wrists, lower yourself down onto your elbows.

tip This exercise is often combined with The Up-stretch (see page 157).

THE FRONT SUPPORT

Start in a push-up position, imagining your body is a plank, with one long line from the crown of your head to your heels. Your shoulders should be directly over your wrists. ①

To align your neck, visualise the heels of your palms as the base of a triangle and your eye-line as the pinnacle of that triangle. Balance on the balls of your feet, keeping them a few inches apart. Hold this position, keeping your buttocks firm and your navel drawn firmly towards your spine, and slowly breathe in and out ten times.

THE LEG PULL FRONT I

Start in a push-up position, imagining your body is a plank, with one long line from the crown of your head to your heels. Your shoulders should be directly over your wrists. ①

Breathe in to prepare.

Maintaining square hips and a still torso, breathe out as you tighten the back of your left thigh and buttock, then point your foot and lift your leg as far as you can. ②

As you breathe in, return to the start position.

Repetitions: Five alternating to each side.

THE LEG PULL FRONT II

Start in a push-up position, imagining your body is a plank, with one long line from the crown of your head to your heels. Your shoulders should be directly over your wrists. ①

Breathe in to prepare.

Keep your buttocks firm and your naval drawn firmly to your spine. Maintaining square hips and a still torso, breathe out as you tighten the back of your left thigh, then point your foot and lift your leg as far as you can. ②

Breathe in and lower your leg until your toes hover just above the floor.

Repetitions: Five on each side.

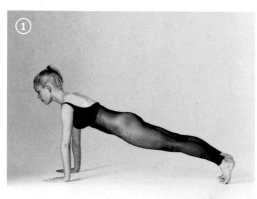

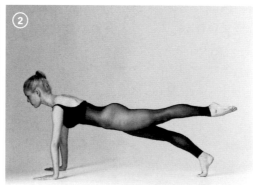

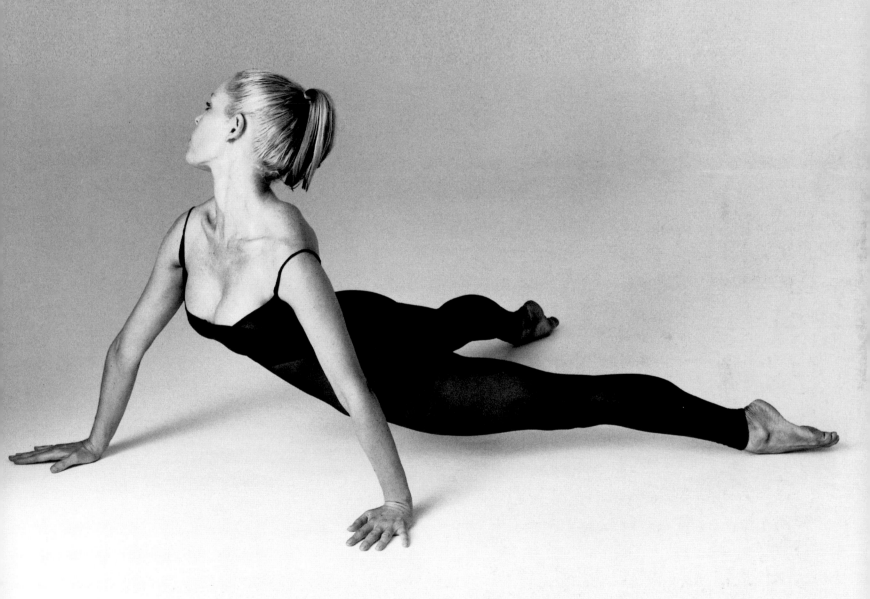

Switching on our body's internal mirror encourages us to take responsibility for our decisions.

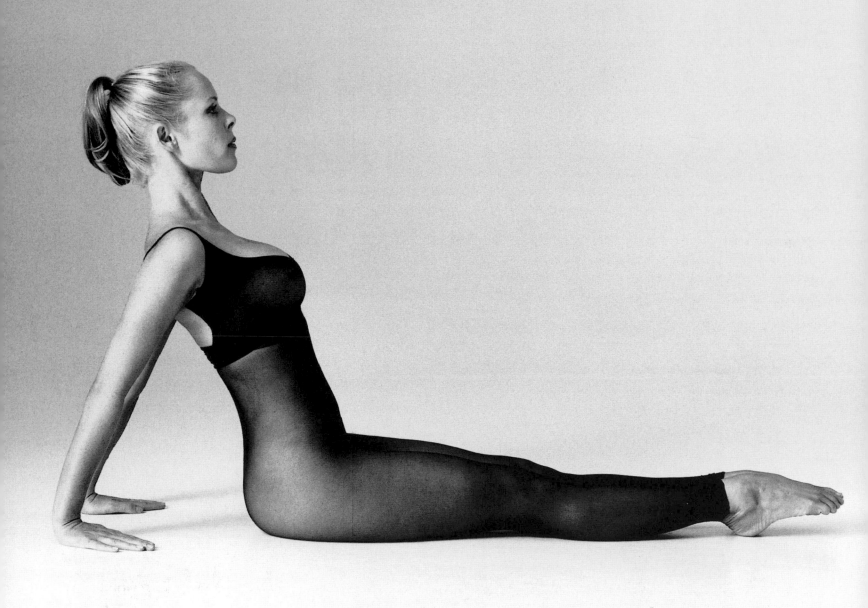

Grace and poise are not gifts we are born with; they are skills that can only be attained through continual practice and precision.

the leg pull back

focus Torso stabilisation and upper-body strength.

imagery Visualise your body in a plank position, with one long line from the crown of your head to your toes.

precaution If you feel any discomfort in your wrists, lower yourself down onto your elbows. If you feel any discomfort in your knees, bend your legs (with a 90-degree angle at the knee joint), with your feet hip-width apart. If you feel any discomfort in your lower back, stop the exercise.

THE BACK SUPPORT

Sit up straight. Place your hands palm-down at least 1 foot behind you, with your fingertips facing towards your hips, and stretch your legs together straight out in front of you. ①

Lift your body into a reverse plank position, visualising one long line from the crown of your head to your toes, being careful to keep your chin slightly lowered and soft, maintaining the alignment with your spine. ②

If you feel any discomfort in your wrists, lower yourself down onto your elbows. If you feel any discomfort in your knees, bend your legs (with a 90-degree angle at the knee joint), with your feet hip-width apart. ③ If you feel any discomfort in your lower back, stop the exercise.

Hold the position as you slowly breathe in and out ten times.

THE LEG PULL BACK I

Sit up straight. Place your hands palm-down at least 1 foot behind you, with your fingertips facing towards your hips, and stretch your legs together straight out in front of you. ① »

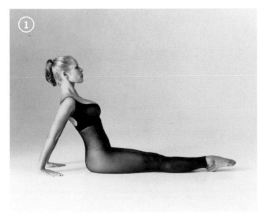

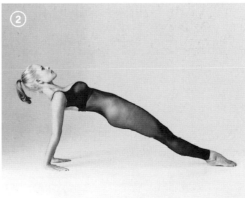

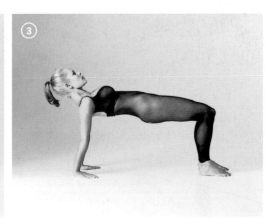

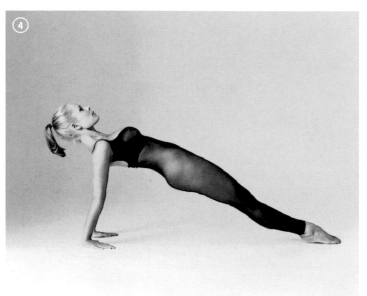

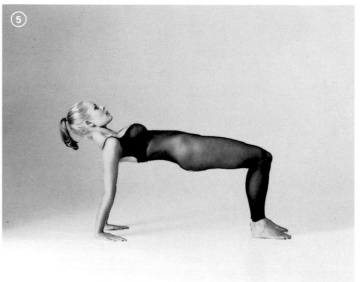

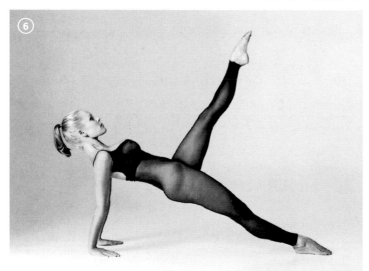

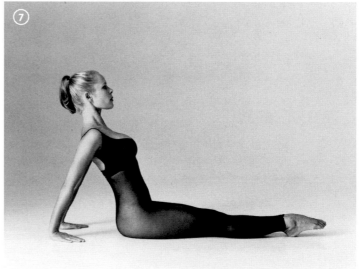

Breathe in to prepare. As you breathe out lift your body into a reverse plank position, visualising one long line from the crown of your head to your toes, being careful to keep your chin slightly lowered and soft, maintaining the alignment with your spine. ④

If you feel any discomfort in your wrists, lower yourself down onto your elbows. If you feel any discomfort in your knees, bend your legs (with a 90-degree angle at the knee joint), with your feet hip-width apart. ⑤ If you feel any discomfort in your lower back, stop the exercise.

Breathe in holding the reverse plank position.

Maintaining square hips and a still torso, breathe out as you tighten the back of your right thigh and buttocks, then point your left foot and lift your leg as high as you can. ⑥

Breathe in and return to the start position.

Repetitions: Five alternating to each side.

THE LEG PULL BACK II

Sit up straight. Place your hands palm-down at least 1 foot behind you, with your fingertips facing towards your hips, and stretch your legs together straight out in front of you. ⑦

Lift your body into a reverse plank position, visualising one long line from the crown of your head to your toes, being careful to keep your chin slightly lowered and soft, maintaining the alignment with your spine. ④

If you feel any discomfort in your wrists, lower yourself down onto your elbows. If you feel any discomfort in your knees, bend your legs (with a 90-degree angle at the knee joint), with your feet hip-width apart. ⑤ If you feel any discomfort in your lower back, stop the exercise.

Breathe in holding the reverse plank position.

Maintaining square hips and a still torso, breathe out as you tighten the back of your right thigh and buttocks, then point your left foot and lift your leg as far as you can. ⑥

Breathe in as you lower your leg until your heel hovers just above the floor.

Repetitions: Five lifting your left leg and then five lifting your right leg.

the side kick kneeling

focus Lateral stabilisation, the sides of your abdominals, balance, control and the outer thigh.

imagery Visualise a sling wrapped underneath your waist holding up your torso.

precaution Stop if you feel any lower-back or knee discomfort.

a s

Kneel on your right knee, keeping your hip directly over your knee. Place your right hand on the floor beside you, with your fingertips pointing away from your body and your shoulder directly above the heel of your palm. Place your left hand behind your head, keeping your elbow open and your shoulder and shoulder blades drawing down your back towards your hip, as you press the heel of your right palm firmly into the floor, lifting up out of your neck and shoulders and stabilising your shoulder girdle. Imagine a sling lifting your waist upwards until there is one long incline from your pelvis to the crown of your head. Draw your navel towards your spine, stabilising your torso, then lift your left

leg up straight out beside you, to hip height, and point your foot.

As you breathe in, flex your left foot and swing your left leg as far forward as you can, keeping your torso still and dissociating your thigh from your pelvis and allowing your leg to pulse once. This quick movement challenges your torso stabilisation and balance.

As you breathe out, squeeze your buttocks, pointing your foot as you swing your leg back, and once again add an extra pulse, keeping your torso still.

Repetitions: Five sets on each side.

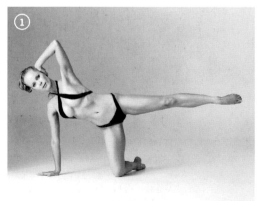

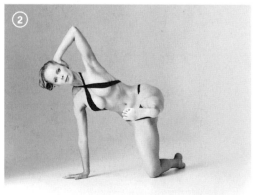

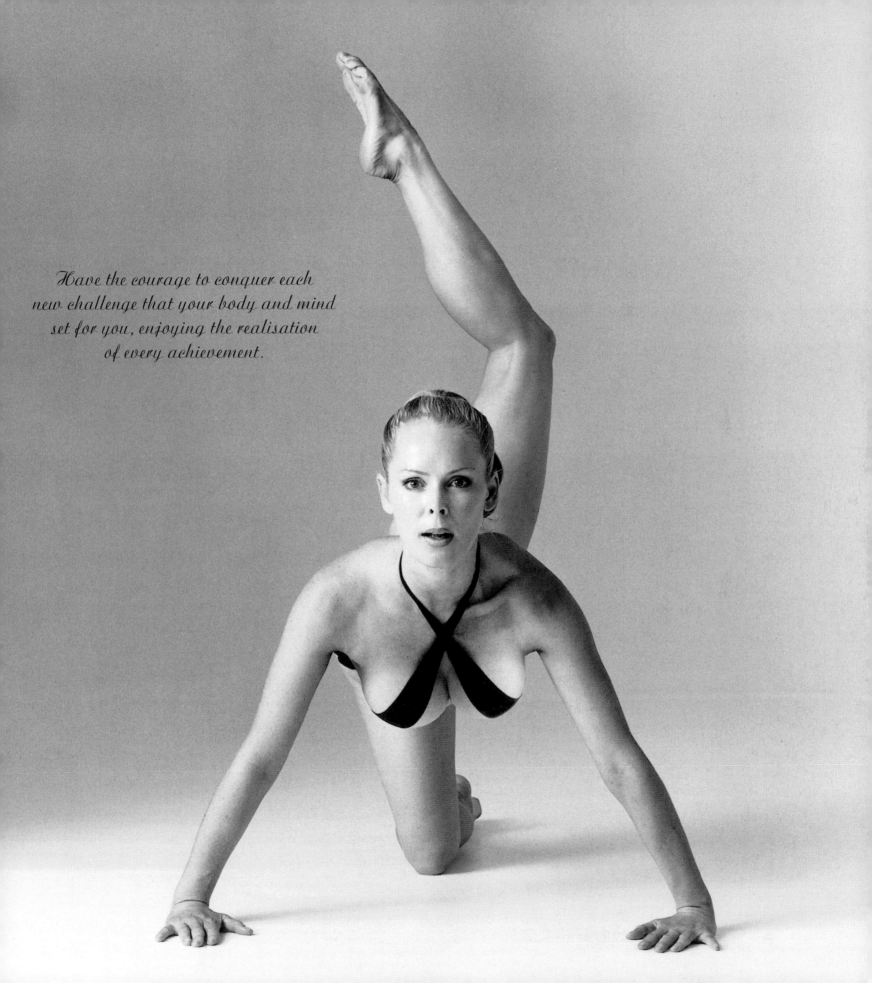

Have the courage to conquer each
new challenge that your body and mind
set for you, enjoying the realisation
of every achievement.

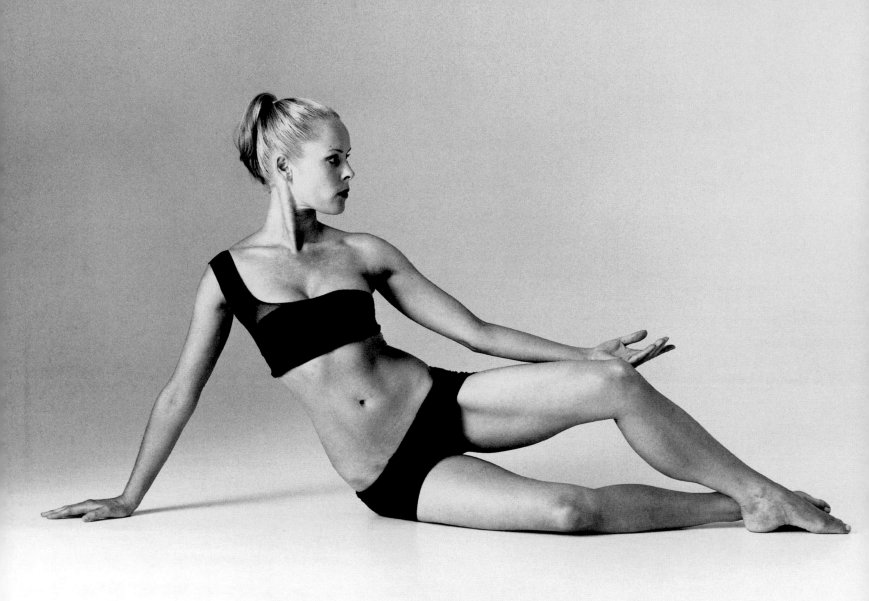

Foresight and planning with our own personal interpretation are the substance of movements that are both beautiful and unique.

the side bend

focus Lateral stabilisation, balance and control, the sides of your abdominals and back.

imagery Visualise your body in a sideways plank, with one long line from the crown of your head to your toes.

precaution Stop if you feel any discomfort in your lower back, shoulder or neck.

Sit on your right hip and place your right hand on the floor beside you, with your fingertips pointing away from your body and the heel of your palm approximately 2 feet away from your shoulder. Stretch your left arm out to the other side at chest height below your shoulder and behind your legs. With your palm facing up and your elbow slightly bent, create a long, flowing curve in your arm, and look towards your left hand. Bend both legs a little and place your left foot in front and flat on the floor, with your kneecap pointing up towards the ceiling. Draw your navel firmly towards your spine, tightening your abdominals. ①

Breathe in to prepare.

As you breathe out, press the heel of your right palm firmly into the floor and shift your shoulder and body weight over your wrist to the right as you lift your body, imagining a sling raising your waist upwards until there is one long incline from the crown of your head to your feet, your left arm lifting to create the letter T, and look down towards your right hand. ②

If you feel any discomfort in your wrists, lower yourself down onto your elbows for the entire exercise. ③

Hold this position as you slowly breathe in and out ten times.

≫

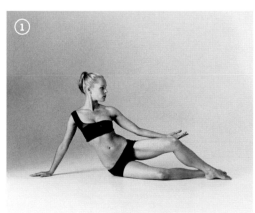

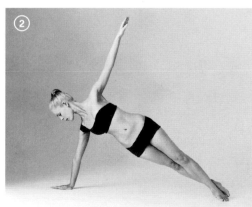

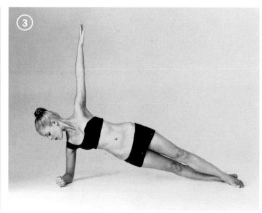

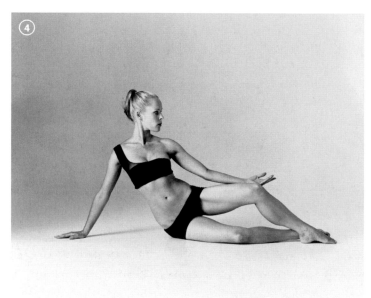

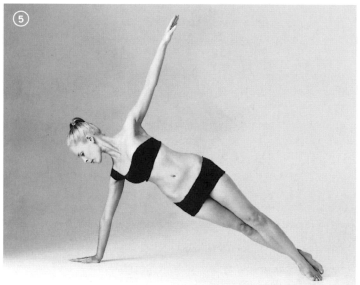

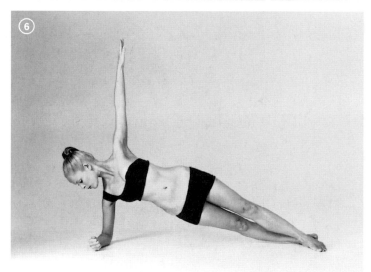

a **s**

Sit on your right hip and place your right hand on the floor beside you, with your fingertips pointing away from your body and the heel of your palm approximately 2 feet away from your shoulder. Stretch your left arm out to the other side at chest height below your shoulder and behind your legs. With your palm facing up and your elbow slightly bent, create a long, flowing curve in your arm, and look towards your left hand. Bend both legs a little and place your left foot in front and flat on the floor, with your kneecap pointing up towards the ceiling. Draw your navel firmly towards your spine, tightening your abdominals. ④

Breathe in to prepare.

As you breathe out, press the heel of your right palm firmly into the floor and shift your shoulder and body weight over your wrist to the right as you lift your body, imagining a sling raising your waist upwards until there is one long incline from the crown of your head to your feet, your left arm lifting to create the letter T, and look towards your right hand. ⑤

If you feel any discomfort in your wrists, lower yourself down onto your elbows for the entire exercise. ⑥

As you breathe in, return to the start position.

Repetitions: Three, then hold the last lift up.

As you breathe in, lower your right hip towards your right wrist until your hip almost touches the floor, keeping your legs straight and visualising your body remaining between two panes of glass. Allow your left arm to lower gracefully in an arc with your palm face-up, and look towards your left hand.

As you breathe out, return to the plank position of your body and the T position of your arm, and look towards your right hand.

Repetitions: Three.

When you have mastered all aspects of this exercise, combine it with The Twist (see page 173) before you change sides.

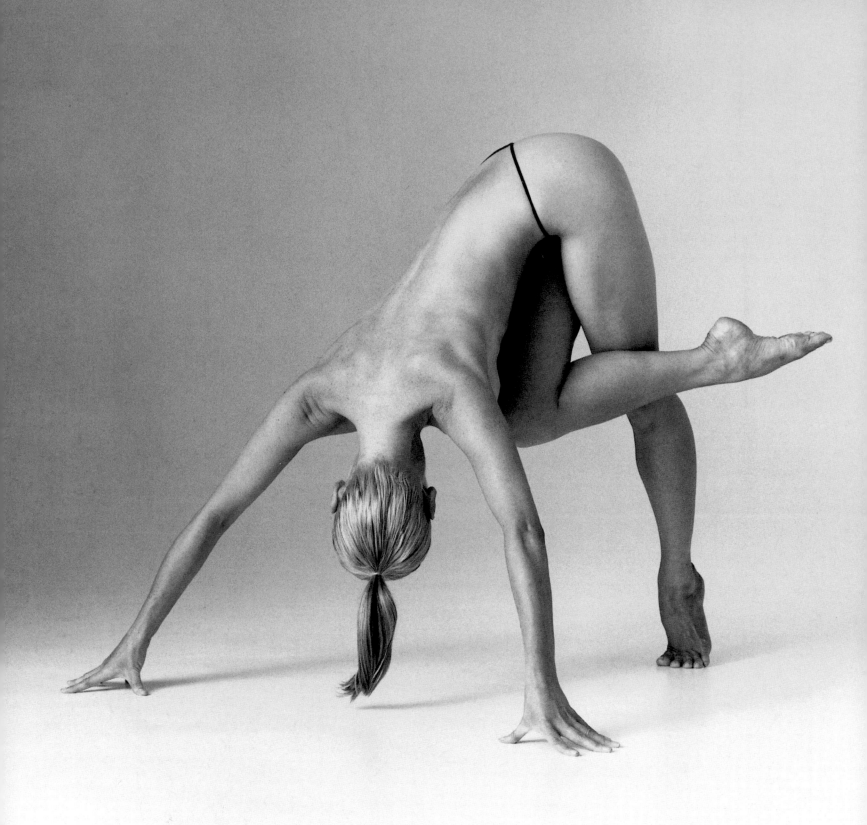

When we challenge ourselves to acquire new skills, we stimulate and nourish our mind, body and spirit.

focus Lateral stabilisation, the sides of your abdominals and back, rotation, balance and control.

imagery Visualise a puppeteer holding a piece of string tied to your tailbone, lifting you straight up towards the ceiling.

precaution Stop if you feel any discomfort in your lower back, shoulders or neck.

a s

This exercise is a continuation of The Side Bend (see page 169), and both should be fully completed on one side before changing to the next.

Sit on your right hip and place your right hand on the floor beside you, with your fingertips pointing away from your body and the heel of your palm approximately 2 feet away from your shoulder. Stretch your left arm out to the other side at chest height below your shoulder and behind your legs. With your palm facing up and your elbow slightly bent, create a long, flowing curve in your arm, and look towards your left hand. Bend both legs a little and place your left foot in front and flat on the floor, with your kneecap pointing up towards

the ceiling. Draw your navel firmly towards your spine, tightening your abdominals.

Breathe in to prepare.

As you breathe out, press the heel of your right palm firmly into the floor and shift your shoulder and body weight over your wrist to the right as you lift your body, imagining a sling raising your waist upwards until there is one long incline from the crown of your head to your feet, your left arm lifting to create the letter T, and look towards your right hand. ②

If you feel any discomfort in your wrists, lower yourself down onto your elbows for the entire exercise. ③ »

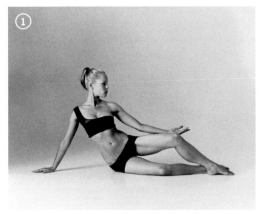

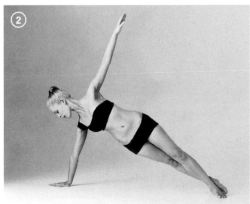

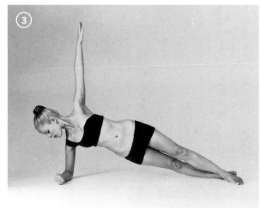

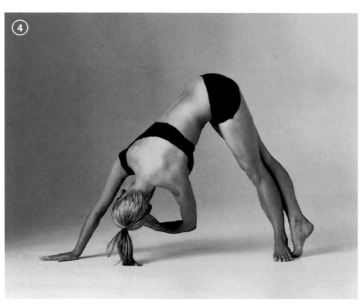

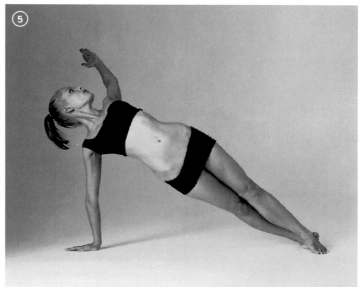

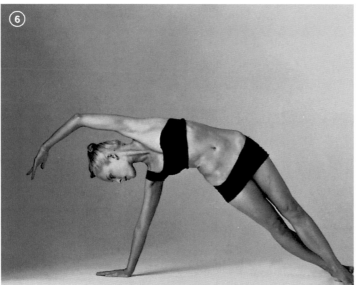

As you breathe in, lift your hips towards the ceiling, creating a reverse V with your body. Threading your left arm through this V, flatten out your spine and look directly behind you. ④

As you breathe out, return to the T position.

As you breathe in, return to the start position.

Repetitions: Three, then hold your final T position.

As you breathe in, allow your upper body to rotate towards the ceiling. Maintaining your balance, take your left arm back and open your chest. ⑤

As you breathe out, return to the T position, carrying your arm over your head.

As you breathe in, lift your ribs closer to the ceiling, creating a graceful arc through your body. ⑥

As you breathe out, return to the T position.

As you breathe in, return to the start position before commencing the other side.

the mermaid

focus Lateral flexion and stretching of the ribs.

imagery Visualise yourself flowing from side to side like a flower swaying in the wind.

precaution If you feel any discomfort in your knee, cross or straighten both legs in front of you.
Stop if you feel any lower-back discomfort.

Sit tall, with your left leg bent behind you and your right leg bent in front of you. Turn your left thigh in from your hip, with your knee heading forward and the inside of your foot facing down. Hold your right inner thigh open, with the inside of your ankle facing up and the sole of your foot in line with your left thigh. Do your best to anchor both sit bones onto the floor equally and stretch both arms out either side of you at chest height, with your palms face-down. ①

Breathe in to prepare.

As you breathe out, bend your right arm and place your elbow and palm down on the floor beside you, and carry your left arm over your head, allowing your palm to softly rotate towards the crown of your head. As you gracefully settle into this pose, imagine a sling wrapped underneath your ribs, drawing your waist up as you press down into your elbow and contract the right side of your abdominals, stretching the left side of your torso. Focus on keeping your left sit bone anchored in this stretch. ②

As you breathe in, return to the start position, reaching your fingertips out to the sides as your spine lengthens up towards the ceiling and your sit bones press down onto the floor.

As you breathe out, hold onto your left knee with your left hand, and sweep your right arm up towards the ceiling, lengthening between each vertebra of your spine, and curve up and over your ribs as you stretch out your right side, allowing your right palm to rotate naturally towards the crown of your head. ③

As you breathe in, return to the start position, reaching your fingertips out to the sides as your spine lengthens up towards the ceiling and your sit bones press down onto the floor.

Repetitions: Three before changing to the other side.

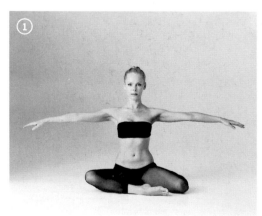

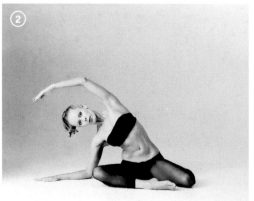

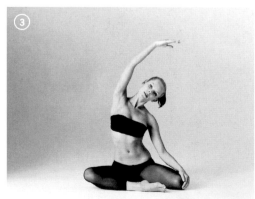

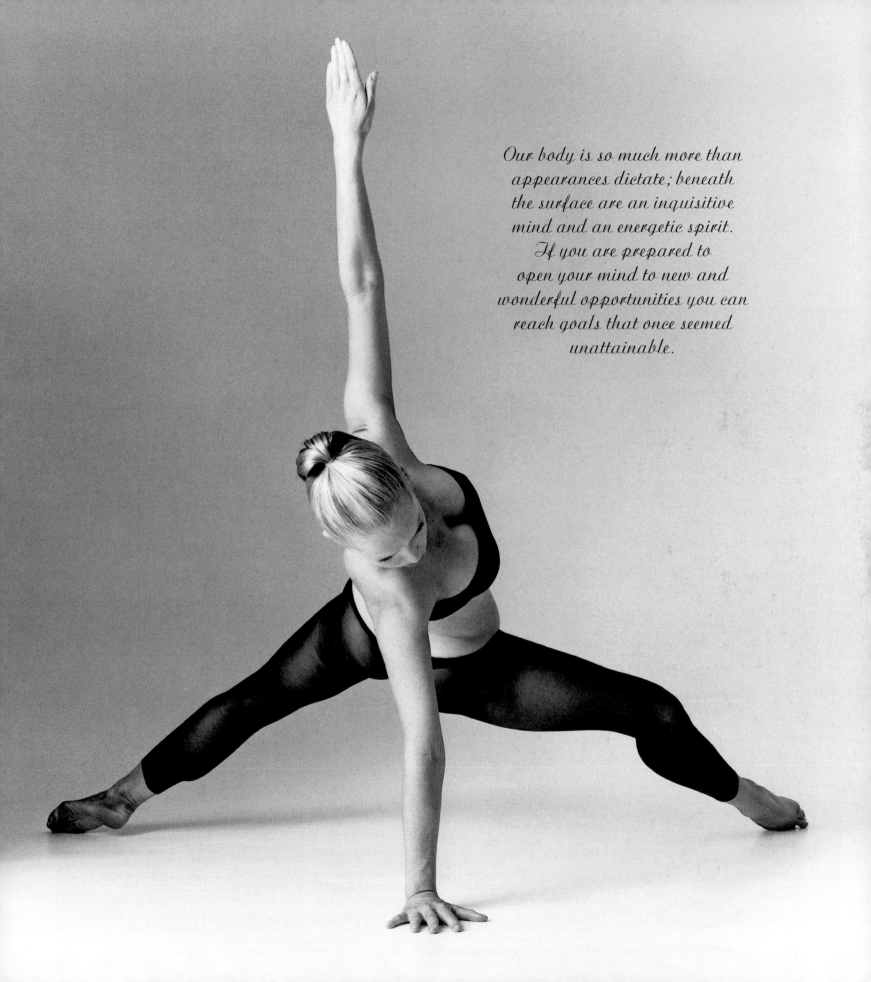

Our body is so much more than
appearances dictate; beneath
the surface are an inquisitive
mind and an energetic spirit.
If you are prepared to
open your mind to new and
wonderful opportunities you can
reach goals that once seemed
unattainable.

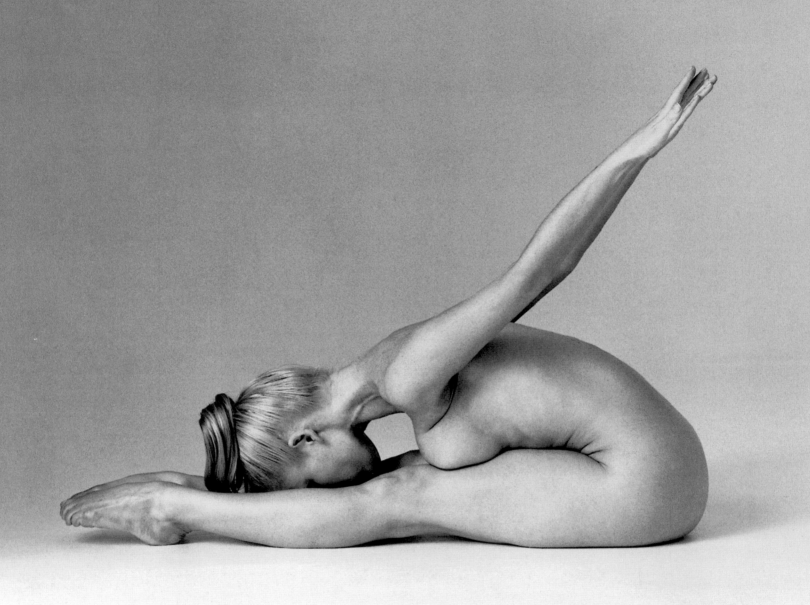

Our body is like a wave in the ocean: constantly changing and adapting to our environment.

the boomerang

focus Balance, control, flowing movement and poise.

imagery Visualise the grace and poise of a ballerina in the role of the dying swan in *Swan Lake*.

Sit with your legs straight out in front of your body, your right ankle crossed over your left and your feet pointed. Drape yourself like the dying swan from the ballet *Swan Lake,* with your chest over your thighs and your arms reaching softly forward, crossing your right wrist over your left. ①

As you breathe in, draw your navel towards your spine and, maintaining a C-curve in your body, start rolling your body backwards, vertebra by vertebra, allowing your hands to slip onto the floor on either side of your legs and slide back along the

floor as you roll backwards and lift your legs. ②

Keeping your hands on the floor beside you, breathe out as you roll back onto the back of your head and shoulders, keeping your body weight between your shoulder blades and off the back of your neck, and sweep your legs backwards over your head, finishing with them behind you parallel to the floor. ③

As you breathe in, change your ankles over in a scissor-like action.

»

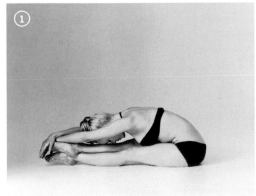

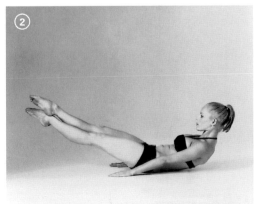

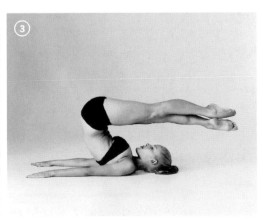

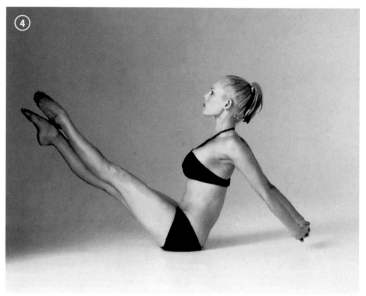

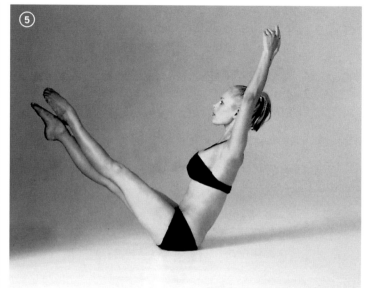

As you breathe out, roll your legs forward over your head and continue rolling until you are in an upright V position, balancing on your tailbone with both legs squeezed together in front and your toes pointed.

As you breathe in, sweep both arms around your body and clasp them behind your back. Open out the front of your chest as you reach your arms as far back as possible in a stretch. ④

Release your clasp as you carry your arms above your head, with your palms facing each other and your shoulders down. ⑤

As you breathe out, simultaneously lower your legs forward with control and reach your arms forward, finishing in the start position with your left ankle and wrist above the right.

Repetitions: Two alternating to each side.

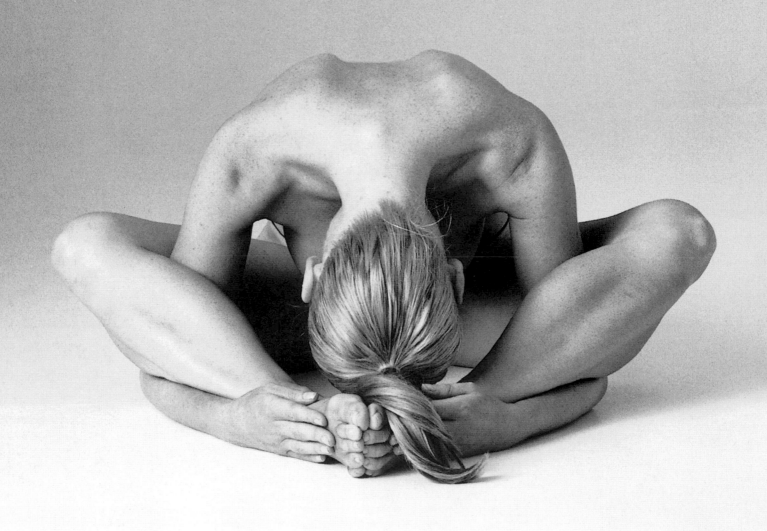

*To appreciate harmony and balance, we sometimes need to apply and experience
two different extremes.*

the seal puppy

focus Balance, control and spinal massage.

imagery Visualise making the shape of a ball with your body.

precaution Ensure your mat is well padded for comfort. Stop the exercise
if you experience any lower-back discomfort.

b

Sit with your spine in a C-curve (shoulders over
hips and navel curved back behind your pelvis),
your legs in a diamond position (knees bent
up and open, big toes touching), your arms
threaded through the centre of your diamond
and your hands wrapped around the front of
your ankles.

Lifting your feet off the floor, lean back
until you find a point of balance behind your
tailbone, finishing with your calves parallel
to the floor.

Maintaining your C-curve, breathe in as you
roll back onto your shoulder blades, keeping
your shoulders, neck and head off the floor,
and your eye-line on your pelvis. ②

As you breathe out, roll back up to the start
position.

Repetitions: Six.

i

Sit up straight, with your legs in a diamond
position (knees bent and open, big toes
touching), your arms threaded through the
centre of your diamond and your hands
wrapped around the front of your ankles.

Maintaining a straight spine, lean back and lift
your feet a few inches off the floor until you find
a point of balance behind your tailbone. ③

»

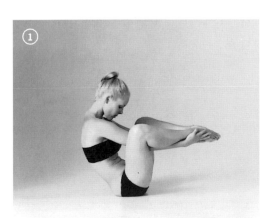

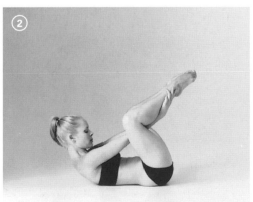

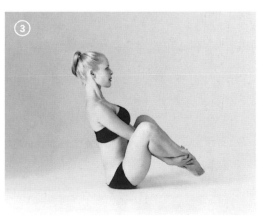

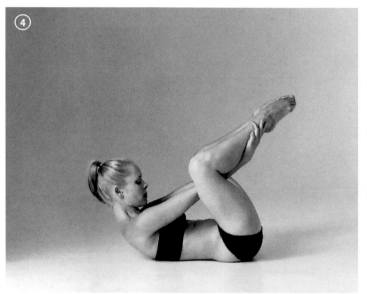

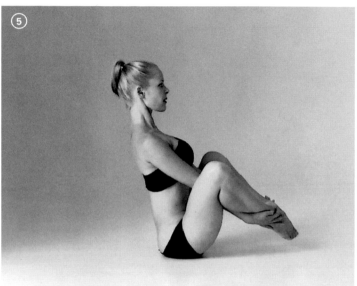

As you breathe in, roll back onto your shoulder blades in a C-curve, keeping your shoulders, neck and head off the floor, and your eye-line on your pelvis. ④

As you breathe out, roll back up to the start position, focusing on using your abdominals to straighten your spine, lengthen your torso and finish with a straight back.

Repetitions: Six.

Sit up straight, your legs in a diamond position (knees bent and open, big toes touching), your arms threaded through the centre of your diamond and your hands wrapped around the front of your ankles.

Maintaining a straight spine, lean back lifting your feet a few inches off the floor until you find a point of balance on your tailbone. ⑤

As you breathe in, roll back onto your shoulder blades in a C-curve, keeping your shoulders, neck and head off the floor, and your eye-line on your pelvis. ④

Holding your balance with your body weight between your shoulder blades, clap your feet together twice like a seal clapping its flippers.

As you breathe out, roll back up to the start position, focusing on using your abdominals to straighten your spine, lengthen your torso and finish with a straight back.

Holding your balance, clap your feet together twice like a seal clapping its flippers.

Repetitions: Six.

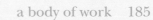

the crab

focus Balance, control and spinal massage.

imagery Visualise making the shape of a ball with your body.

precaution Ensure your mat is well padded for comfort. Stop the exercise
if you experience lower-back discomfort.

Sit with your spine in a C-curve (shoulders over hips and navel curved back behind your pelvis) and your eye-line on your pelvis. Lean back and lift your feet off the floor until you find a point of balance behind your tailbone, hugging your knees, slightly apart, into your chest. Keep the heels of your feet as close to your buttocks as possible, and hold onto the front of your ankles, with your right ankle crossed over the left.

Maintaining your C-curve, breathe in as you roll back onto your shoulder blades. ① Finish with your shoulders, neck and head gently on the floor, and your eye-line still on your pelvis.

Straighten your legs over your head until they finish parallel to the floor and your body weight is balanced between your shoulder blades.

Swap your ankles over.

As you breathe out, bend your legs, keeping the heels of your feet as close to your buttocks as possible, and roll back up to the start position, holding onto the front of your ankles (your left ankle in front of the right).

Continuing forward, breathe in as you balance the crown of your head on the floor, gently stretching the back of your neck, and place your weight on your knees as you lift your ankles and shins off the floor. Squeeze your legs tightly in towards your buttocks. ②

As you breathe out, return to the start position, with your left ankle in front.

Repetitions: Six, alternating the ankle in front each time.

 variation

Instead of finding a balance on the crown of your head as you roll up, continue breathing out as you lower your ankles and knees down onto the floor, releasing your hands and placing them forward on the floor, just to the sides of your knees.

As you breathe in, transfer your weight onto your knees and kneel up. Sweep both arms forward up towards the ceiling and then out to the sides as you look up and lean back slightly, opening your chest as if you were throwing autumn leaves. ③

As you breathe out, sit back down, placing your body weight once more on your hands to assist you back to the original start position.

Repetitions: Six, alternating the ankle in front each time.

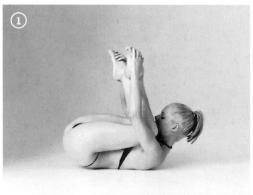

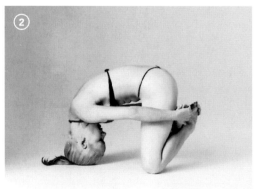

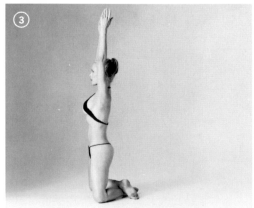

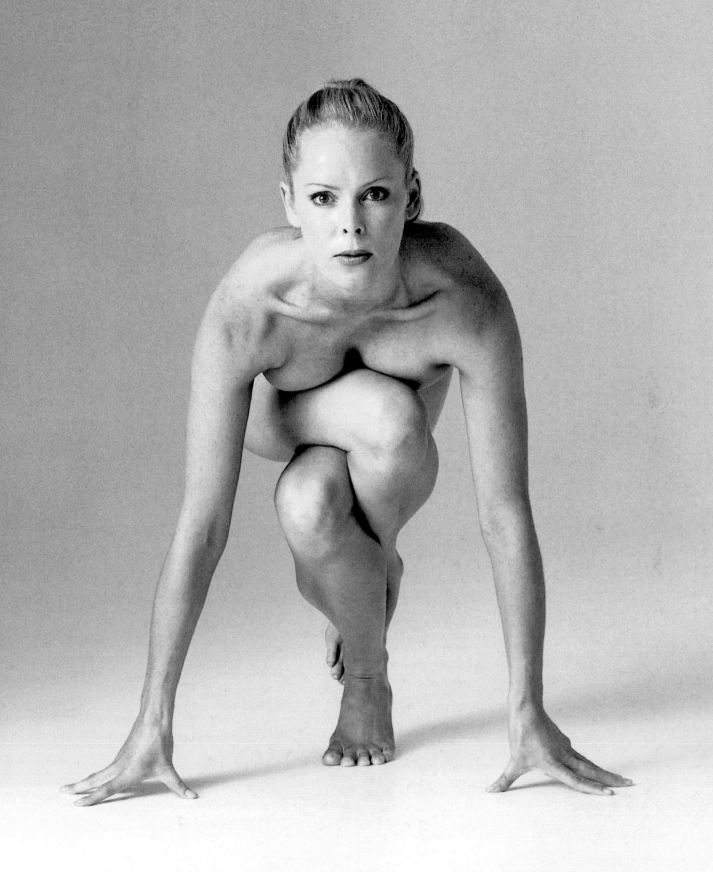

Ultimate concentration is the acceptance of total distraction and the ability to quiet the mind.

the rocking

focus Spine extension, abdominals, shoulder stretch and balance.

imagery Visualise your body moving in the fluid movement of a rocking horse.

precaution If you feel any lower-back discomfort, stop the exercise and move into The Rest Position (see page 108) to release your spine. It is inappropriate to attempt this exercise if you have a neck, shoulder or lower-back issue. This exercise should be performed for the first time under experienced supervision.

Lie face-down, with your head resting on the floor to the right, as if you were listening to the floor. Bend your knees behind you and hold onto the front of your ankles. ①

As you breathe in, lift and open your chest, reaching your toes up towards the ceiling. ②

As you breathe out, return to the start position with your head resting on the floor to the left.

Repetitions: Five.

As you breathe in, lift and open your chest, allowing your neck to follow the natural line

of your spine. Still holding your ankles, reach your arms back and lengthen your toes up towards the ceiling.

As you breathe out, roll forward onto your chest, keeping your head poised and in line with your neck and spine. Focus on initiating this movement from the point at the base of your sternum, simultaneously reaching your toes as far away from your knees as possible.

Breathe in and rock back the other way.

Repetitions: Ten.

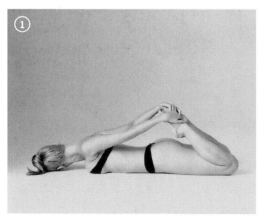

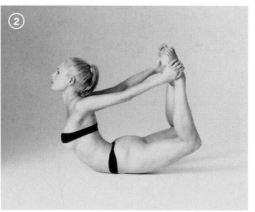

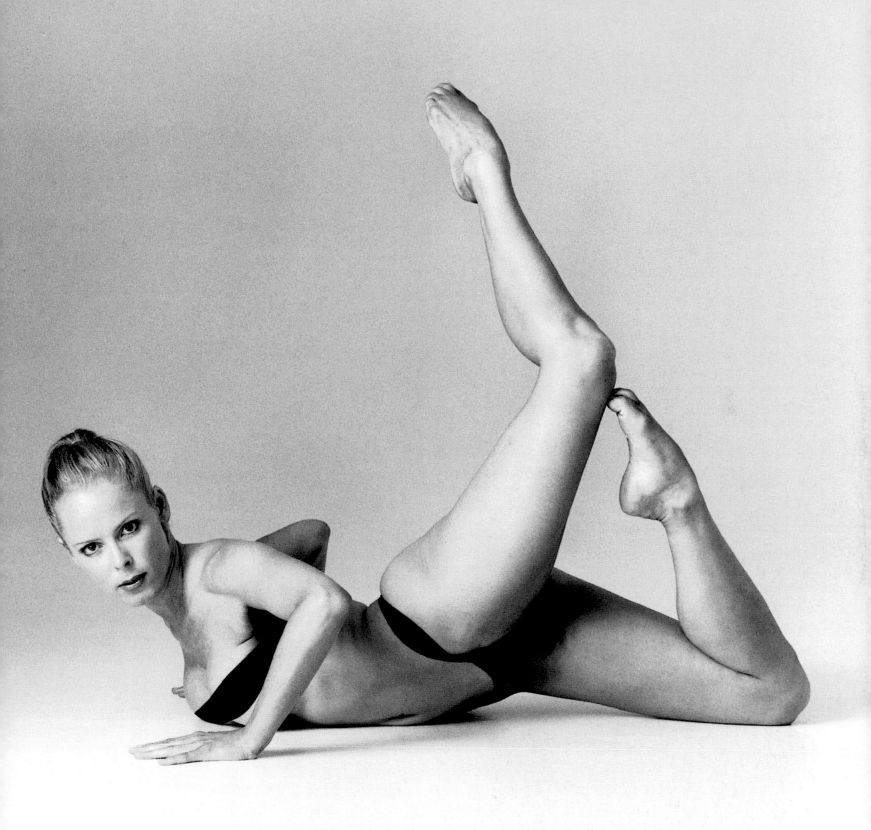

When you realise you are faced with a new and daunting challenge, focus on the smaller goals that need to be realised to conquer your ultimate goal with courage and dignity.

the control balance

focus Balance, control and flowing movement.

imagery Visualise your legs moving smoothly like a pair of scissors.

precaution It is inappropriate to attempt this exercise if you have a neck, shoulder or lower-back issue. This exercise should be performed for the first time under experienced supervision.

Lie on your back, with your arms by your sides, your knees lifted in a tabletop position (90 degrees at hip and knee) and squeezed together and your feet pointed. Drawing your navel towards your spine and anchoring your tailbone, extend your legs straight up.

Breathe in to prepare.

As you breathe out, focus on using your abdominals to carry your legs over your head until they finish parallel to the floor and your body weight is balanced between your shoulder blades. Keep your arms strongly imprinted on the floor beside you. ①

As you breathe in, lower your toes down to the floor behind you and sweep your arms around your sides and back to hold onto your feet. ②

Breathe out percussively, keeping both legs lengthened as you lift your left leg straight up towards the ceiling, squeezing your buttocks and pulsing your leg once quickly as it reaches its highest point, challenging your stability and balance. ③

As you breathe in, change your legs over, timing the split precisely so as to maintain your balance and form.

Repetitions: Five alternating to each side.

As you breathe in, bring your legs together over your head, with your toes touching the floor. Hold firmly onto your ankles as you squeeze your thighs towards your chest.

As you breathe out, roll your spine back down, vertebra by vertebra, keeping your legs squeezed tightly, stretching out the back of your thighs and spine. Release your legs as your tailbone makes contact with the floor, and finish in the start position.

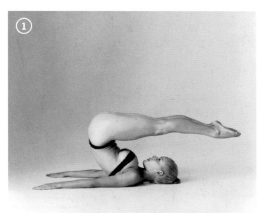

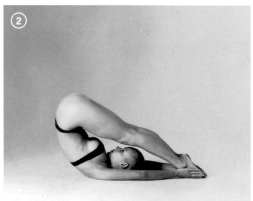

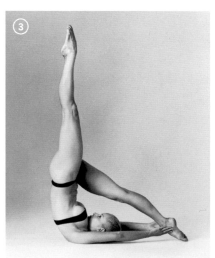

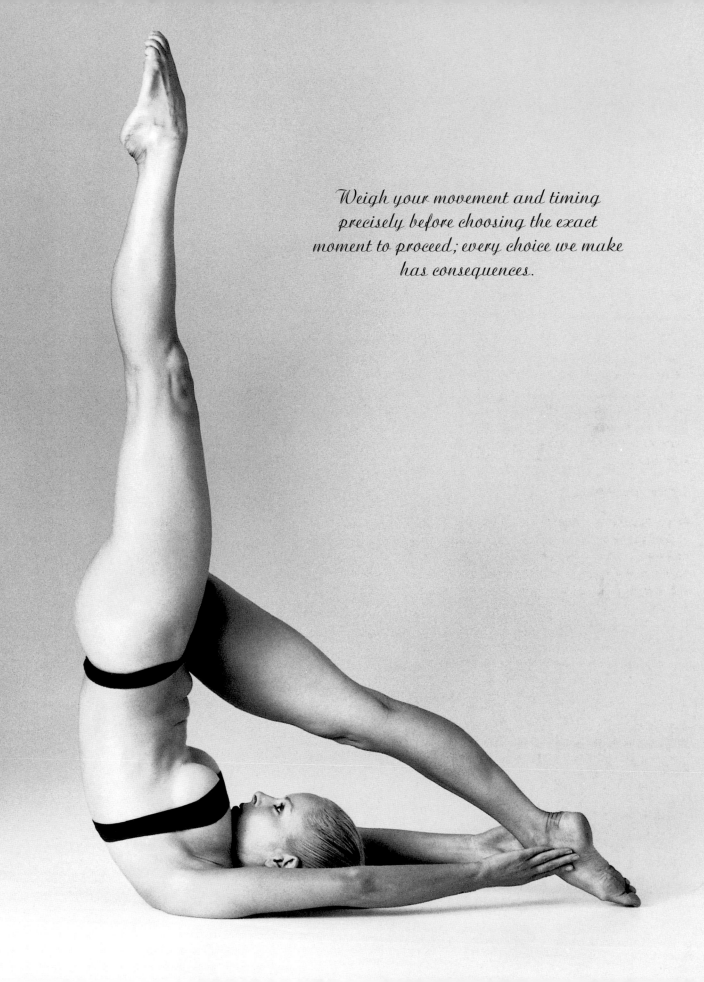

Weigh your movement and timing
precisely before choosing the exact
moment to proceed; every choice we make
has consequences.

the push-up

focus Core conditioning, spinal articulation, hamstring stretch and chest strength.

imagery Visualise a sling wrapped underneath your waist holding up your torso.

precaution Stop if you feel any lower-back, shoulder or wrist discomfort.

Stand tall, visualising a piece of string tied to the crown of your head and being pulled straight up into the sky like a puppet string, encouraging you to be your tallest. Relax your arms down by your side, soften your knees and separate your feet slightly in a parallel alignment with your knees.

Breathe in to prepare.

As you breathe out, lower your chin, soften your chest and roll your spine forward vertebra by vertebra, as if you were peeling yourself off a sticky wall. Keeping your neck and shoulders relaxed, roll all the way down to the floor and place your hands on the floor in front of you. If you feel tightness in the back of your thighs or spine, bend your legs until you are comfortable.

As you breathe in, walk your hands forward and press your heels down into the floor, stretching out the back of your calves and thighs, and finish with your body in the shape of a pyramid, your shoulders drawing down your back toward your hips. Imagine that you now have a straight line running up from the heels of your palms to your tailbone and a straight line from your tailbone down to your heels. ①

Keeping your heels as low as possible, breathe out as you transfer your body into a plank position, imagining you have one long line from the crown of your head to your heels. The heels of your palms should be lined up with the middle of your ribs. To align your neck, visualise the heels of your palms as the base of a triangle and your eye-line as the pinnacle of that triangle. ②

As you breathe in, bend your elbows, keeping them close to your sides, and keep your chest and upper back broad, maintaining a long neck and firm abdominals. ③

As you breathe out, straighten your arms.

As you breathe in, return to the pyramid position, and walk your hands back towards your feet, once again bending your knees if necessary.

As you breathe out, roll your spine back up, vertebra by vertebra, and return to the start position.

Repetitions: Up to ten. (Build each repetition progressively. For example, do one push-up for the first repetition, then two push-ups for the second repetition, and so on.)

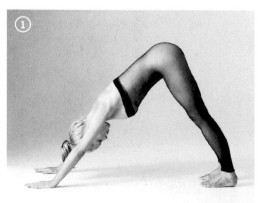

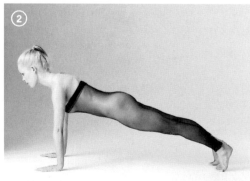

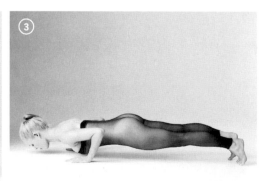

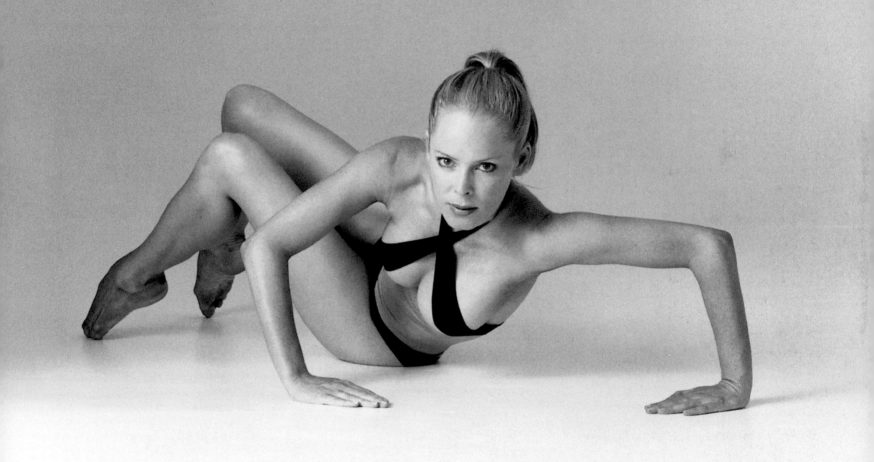

Focusing totally on the moment is a form of meditation; it is grounding.

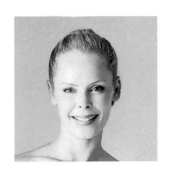

A former professional ballerina, Helen Tardent discovered Pilates while studying at The Royal Ballet School in London. After retiring from the world of dance in 1992 Helen brought her passion for Pilates to Australia. In 1998 Helen launched the first Pilates Matwork classes in an Australian gym and then, in 2000, she opened the Pilates Moves studio at Double Bay, Sydney, where she offers a broad range of individual and group classes, and also launched group Reformer classes in Australia for the first time.

Since 2001 Helen has hosted the Pilates shows on *Aerobics Oz Style*, a weekday television program aired in forty countries worldwide. As an important member of the Australian Pilates community, Helen travels throughout Australia training hundreds of instructors each year.

In 2003 Helen co-founded the Mind Your Body conference, drawing together the widespread Pilates, Yoga and associated modalities and allowing health professionals to further their education in a positive, non-competitive environment.

Helen Tardent's personal goal and vision is to provide quality instructor training and introduce the Pilates Method of Exercise, the dance industry's best-kept secret, to the general public.

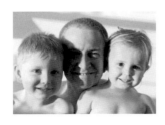

Greg Barrett has worked extensively in Performing Arts photography. His clients include the Australian Ballet, Bangarra, the Australian Chamber Orchestra and Opera Australia. He has produced two previous photography books on dance, *Danceshots* and the best-selling *tutu*, made in collaboration with the dancers of The Australian Ballet, and has directed over 450 short films and television commercials.

Prints of Greg's photographic work are collected privately and publicly and The National Library in Canberra holds many of Greg's portraits in its permanent collection.

Greg is married with two children and is currently living and working in New York.

acknowledgements

My family, I cherish my upbringing and each individual's input that has been instrumental in my life's goals.

Rael Isacowitz, you were instrumental in firing my passion for Pilates and you inspired me to share this passion with the world.

Sandy Sellers, your enthusiasm, creativity and inner beauty is an inspiration to me.

Stan Barnes, my dearest friend, just thinking of you invokes the peace and tranquillity I feel in your presence.

Paul Driscoll, your second opinion and humorous reasoning have always been of such value in all my important decisions before they became realities! Your significant input into my professional journey has become a remarkable friendship.

Genia Lifschitz, my very own JM, I can't imagine what my life would be like without your smile and guidance.

Greg Barrett, simple words fail to express the inspiration I had working with such a beautiful soul.

Guy Lawrence, you're a genius with my hair and very brave for being present for the entire photo shoot!

Sandy Wagner, without your encouragement this book would still be a dream.

Julie Gibbs, your extraordinary passion for publishing and life is beautiful. I feel privileged to be a part of your vision.

Claire de Medici, my editor, I really appreciate how involved you kept me through the entire process; it was an incredible and exciting experience.

Melissa Fraser, my designer, watching you create the reality of my dream was an awesome experience.

index

This book is not intended to replace or supersede professional medical advice. The advice and exercises in this book are intended to complement professional Pilates classes taught by a qualified Pilates instructor. Neither the author nor the publisher may be held responsible for claims resulting from information contained in this book.

LANTERN

Published by the Penguin Group
Penguin Group (Australia)
250 Camberwell Road, Camberwell, Victoria 3124, Australia
(a division of Pearson Australia Group Pty Ltd)
Penguin Group (USA) Inc.
375 Hudson Street, New York, New York 10014, USA
Penguin Group (Canada)
10 Alcorn Avenue, Toronto, Ontario, Canada M4V 3B2
(a division of Pearson Penguin Canada Inc.)
Penguin Books Ltd
80 Strand, London WC2R 0RL, England
Penguin Ireland
25 St Stephen's Green, Dublin 2, Ireland
(a division of Penguin Books Ltd)
Penguin Books India Pvt Ltd
11 Community Centre, Panchsheel Park, New Delhi – 110 017, India
Penguin Group (NZ)
Cnr Airborne and Rosedale Roads, Albany, Auckland, New Zealand
(a division of Pearson New Zealand Ltd)
Penguin Books (South Africa) (Pty) Ltd
24 Sturdee Avenue, Rosebank, Johannesburg 2196, South Africa

Penguin Books Ltd, Registered Offices: 80 Strand, London, WC2R 0RL, England

First published by Penguin Group (Australia), a division of Pearson Australia Group Pty Ltd, 2005

10 9 8 7 6 5 4 3 2 1

Text copyright © Helen Tardent 2005
Photographs copyright © Greg Barrett 2005

Design by Melissa Fraser © Penguin Group (Australia)
Photography by Greg Barrett
Typeset in News Gothic by Post Pre-press Group and Melissa Fraser
Printed and bound in China through Bookbuilders

National Library of Australia
Cataloguing-in-Publication data:

Tardent, Helen.
Beautiful Pilates.

Includes index.
ISBN 1 920989 11 0.

1. Pilates method. 2. Health. I. Title.

613.71

www.penguin.com.au